Sirtfood Diet

Complete Step-by-Step Guide to Cooking Healthy Dishes and Losing Weight Quickly with the Sirtfood Diet

Shanon Hope Caldwell

Table of Content

Introduction

This book would be a guide for people who want to lose weight quickly and who are interested in new trends. It is for the people who would like to learn more about the science behind sirtuin protein, how it works, why it's different from other diets, and how people can eat what they enjoy like chocolate and wine without getting scammed by promises. Success Stories of celebrities who tried and used this diet to lose weight are also included. I am talking about sirtfoods diet. It has been adopted by many people, including Pippa Middleton, Lorraine Pascale, the Food Network Chef, the actress Jodi Kidd, Sir Ben Ainslie, and a boxer named David Haye. Sirt foods help signal your body to restore your metabolism and increase muscle mass while burning fat. You will stay energetic, besides losing extra fats because sirtfood contain a bundle of green vegetables and juice that will keep your stomach full. The list of sirt foods include kale, celery, walnuts, Red wine, Strawberries, Onions, Soy, Parsley, Extra virgin olive oil, Dark chocolate (85% cocoa), Matcha green tea, Buckwheat, Turmeric, Arugula (rocket), Bird's eye chili, Lovage, Medjool dates, Red chicory, Blueberries, Capers and Coffee. You do not have to leave your chocolates, and red wine will also be on your menu. You can make delicious recipes for breakfast, lunch, dinner including drinks, salads, fried and foods along with desserts. You can make recipes like sirt muesli, coronated chicken, baked potatoes, chocolate sirtfood bites, kale and blackcurrant smoothies and many more. Include these recipes in your life and take it as your lifestyle not as a diet. You will enjoy your fat loss journey by following the meal plans of sirtfood diet phases and maintain it to live smarter.

Chapter 1: Sirtfood Basics

There is a whole range of diets there to choose from, but it's all about doing what is right for you. The sirtfood diet, eating program stars like Adele and Pippa Middleton swear by, is one of the latest to gain popularity. Let's go through exactly what the sirtfood diet is, before you start trying it out for yourself.

1.1 What is Sirtfood Diet?

The sirtfood diet works off the idea that you can cause activation of certain proteins called sirtuins or descriptively dubbed "skinny genes" by eating certain items. Sirtfood Diet was created by two celebrity nutritionists Aidan Goggins and Glen Matten working for a private gym in the UK. They promote the diet as a revolutionary new diet and health program that works by turning the "skinny gene" on. Some natural plant compounds may increase the level of these proteins in the body, and the foods they contain have been dubbed "sirt foods." The diet guarantees that in seven days you will lose 7lbs and the weight loss will not be muscle, not fat. They 're all tasty and easy to add to your diet. All these have in common are natural plant chemicals called polyphenols that are responsible for sirtuin genes being turned on. The polyphenols in plants help them to adjust to the challenges of their environment. When we eat plants with polyphenols, our stress-response pathways are triggered and can mimic the effects of fasting and exercise by doing just that: fasting and exercise. Although all plants have an inbuilt system to react to environmental stressors, only a select few can generate significant amounts of polyphenols triggered by sirtuin. These are the foods made with sirts.

1.2 What are Skinny Genes and Do the Diet Influence Skinny Genes Activation?

Over the years, numerous clinical experiments have been performed to better decide whether there are indeed "skinny genes". How do some people struggle with their weight while others appear for eating what they want without gaining on any extra weight? Though diet and lifestyle are the distinct contributing factors, weight variations in animals have given us reason to think there might be more to it than that; and perhaps there's even more of an internal driving force-genes. Throughout the years, up to 50 different genes are found and also thought to affect our weight and body composition. Many of these are considered to change how we digest and metabolize fats, and also affect our appetite.

One of the most current findings was the "skinny gene "which has been so-called "adipose". This was initially discovered in fruit flies, but has also been observed in rodents and humans. If this gene is turned on, the individual is more likely to be "skinny", in comparison to if it's switched off we're more likely to store more fat or adipose tissue. However, interestingly the "skinny gene" isn't thought to switched on or off, but can be switched on to various degrees in different people.

While people are becoming more interested in genetics and what genes we can or not have – the fact is you're stuck with your genetic makeup. However, what I also want to pay focus is that you can affect these genes in a variety of ways:

The Power of Nutrition Can Turn off and On to Skinny Genes.

We know that diet and our environment will affect our genes directly. Interestingly the 'skinny gene 'is believed to be turned on to varying degrees in different individuals – because everybody has it, we need to control it.

Genetic Factors are not the Whole Thing that Matters

Although certain people may be disposed to certain things as a result of their genes, whenever we talk about the bodyweight (and many of other factors like disease states), there are numerous of reasons to believe that we can manage even genes, as a result of external influences like diet and lifestyle, at least to a specific extent! For the vast majority of people, monitoring their diet or focusing on more exercise would have the desired impact when performed in the right way.

Do not Blame Genes for Your Obesity

We are just blaming our genes risks being a bit of a cop-out when it comes to body weight. As both obesity and the associated diseases such as diabetes have increased exponentially in all parts of the world over a similar time frame in recent years, we know that genes aren't the whole story. This trend suggests diet, eating habits, and social influences are much more likely to be playing the leading role.

Is there some Specific Diet to Turn On Skinny Genes?

There seems to be a relentless influx of new fad diets available nowadays, and it can be challenging to know which, if any of them, are likely to be appropriate for promoting your wellbeing or particular weight loss goals. In terms of possibly affecting specific 'skinny genes,' the Sirtfood Diet has gained some special attention recently. The Sirtfood Diet is so-called as it is rich in foods high in unique chemical compounds called sirtuin activators. Sirtuins are a specific class of enzymes which are thought to have beneficial effects in the body.

1.3 What are Sirtuins and What is the Science behind Them?

Some fads, frauds and quackery profoundly are corrupting few items as nutrition. As such, it is through a prism of healthy scepticism that we should consider every new diet. The latest update these days is the Sirtfood diet which, if we take claims, will assist with weight loss as well as providing other benefits such as "stimulating rejuvenation and cellular repair". To the uninitiated, this latest diet is focused on consumption of foods which will interact with a proteins family known as sirtuin proteins or SIRT1-SIRT7. By adding to the diet's undoubted appeal is the fact that the best sources consist of red wine and chocolate, as well as citrus fruits, blueberries and kale.

The sirtuin firstly was found in yeast and was called the information regulation or sirt2 or the silent pairing type. It is the gene that's responsible for yeast cell regeneration. Sirtuins are a signaling protein family that is involved in metabolic regulation. They are ancient in animal evolution and appear to have a structure that is highly conserved in all areas of life. In complex mammals, seven enzymes are known. And what do we think about the diet? The response from a scientific point of view is: in response to changes in energy levels, sirtuins contribute to the regulation of fat and glucose metabolism. Also, they could play a role in the effect of calorie restriction on ageing improvements. It may be through the implications of sirtuins on aerobic (or mitochondrial) metabolism, decreasing species of reactive oxygen (free radicals), and increasing antioxidant enzymes.

Sirtuin 1-7 belongs to the third class of deacetylase enzymes, and for its action is dependent on NAD+. Sirtuin modulation can potentially have a positive impact on human diseases, leading to a growing interest in small molecules that change their activity, according to recent studies. It caused an uproar in sirtuin and sirtuin activator research. Sirt 1-7 is responsible for benefits such as DNA repair, growth, inflammation, regulation of metabolism, stable ageing, neuroprotection, apoptosis and survival of cells. Each sirtuin shall be responsible for their associated gain. Sirt1 has been the most studied phenomenon so far since it comes nearest to Sirt2.

Sirt1 regulates the metabolism, Sirt1's activity is governed by the body's nutritional status, which it up-regulates during calorie reduction. Mammalian studies indicate that deletion of sirt2 can be the cause of tumor growth, suggesting that sirt2 can be responsible for the suppression of tumor. Sirt3 has shown in research that it can theoretically prolong the lifespan of humans. Sirt4 is accountable for the production of insulin and may have a metabolic function. Although sirt5 is known to detoxify ammonia, sirt6 has remarkable properties and is recommended for cancer therapy due to its essential role in restoring DNA. Sirt7 is responsible for controlling the transcription of rRNA. Sirtuins get activated in conjunction with nicotinamide adenine dinucleotide or NAD +. NAD is a critical factor in metabolism and occurs in every living cell. Sirtuin depends on NAD + being activated. And without NAD +, the Sirtuin will avoid doing something.

Limiting calories and speed is one of the most effective and well-known ways of activating sirtuins and autophagy. It will signal to the body that it is in a survival scenario and has to activate these genes for longevity. Sirtuin-activating compounds (STACs) are compounds that affect sirtuins and mimic the restriction of calories.

They can slow down ageing and avoid age-related diseases such as Alzheimer's. Resveratrol is thought to imitate caloric restraint by triggering SIRT1. Those claims were disputed, though, and are dependent on other background paths. However, resveratrol has also been found to imitate caloric restriction, despite many of its benefits such as decreased oxidative stress, lower inflammation, enhanced cardiovascular function and increased cognition[lii]. Resveratrol can inhibit mTOR and activate AMPK, which has longevity benefits similar to sirtuins.

- Sirtuins may be modulated by polyphenols found in bitter vegetables, olive oil, dark chocolate, curcumin, ginger, ginseng and dark berries. There are polyphenols in coffee and teas too. The Nrf2 pathway is activated by coffee, broccoli and spices, which can cause the antioxidant defense effect.
- Curcumin stimulates SIRT1 and prevents the Beta-amyloid plaque neurotoxicity found in Alzheimer's[lv]. Ginger,

Cinnamon and Turmeric are an integral part of my daily antioxidant use.

- With many antioxidant benefits, quercetin is the most commonly used flavonoid in the human diet[xiv] and activates SIRT1. Elderberries, red onions, hot peppers, cranberries, kale, and tomatoes are included. Catechins, quercetin, butein, fisetin, and kaempferol are also compounds found to increase sirtuins in the same foods.

- DHA raises SIRT1 and enhances blood vessel function and cerebral flow. Fatty fish, eggs, and algae are the best sources of DHA.

- Zinc is essential for maintaining operation on SIRT1. Zinc can be found in meat, fish, and seafood. These foods, however, also increase mTOR signaling, which can counterbalance sirtuin effects.

- Nicotinamide Riboside (NR) is an NAD+ precursor that assists in the metabolism of carbon. It's also a source of vitamin B3 contained in raw dairy supplements such as yeast, mushrooms or niacin. It could support shuttle to SIRT1.

Add the Sirtfood Diet Plan in Your Life

Instead of following a super-strict routine and prescriptive recipes, why not just attempt to include some of the Sirtfood diet components into your diet anyway? Whether the sirtuins have specific actions in the body or not, these foods are packed with vitamins, minerals and antioxidants that are important to support healthy body processes and a buzzing metabolism. I firmly believe that fresh-cooking is the secret to healthy body weight. It's all the refined foods with secret sugars, salts, fat (and the rest!) that contribute even more to piling us on the pounds. Eat new, get into your meal preparation and cooking routines, and you'll soon feel the difference and note it.

Instead of Genes Change Your Nutrition Pattern

There's almost nothing you can't do to influence your genes, even the experts have agreed. So even though we're predisposed to other forms of body or disease disorders, that means we 're at a higher risk of these various states, it's not unavoidable that we'll get affected. So our diet, everyday habits and aspects of lifestyle can all have an impact, and even minor adjustments could make a difference for the planet. One top tip to consider is the amount of water you 're drinking.

We know that water affects every system in our body, and research has suggested that this pure constituent of our diet might be crucial to supporting our genes and overall health. Not only are there the benefits of drinking, but you are less likely to drink other things if you drink more water-even potentially more dangerous things.

Recently, there is a constant increase in the consumption of calorific drinks, and with calories all the sugar, artificial sweeteners, caffeine and alcohol that are common components of drinks that are not water – all of which are unlikely to do any favors to your metabolism! So, drink, and add a slice of lemon or some other fruit if you first struggle. More of sirt drinks recipes are shared in the coming chapters in details for you. By trying those recipes, you will be able to have more water intake in various forms.

Chapter 2: Sirtfood Diet and Research

2.1 Some Examples from the Past about Losing their Weight with Sirtfood

Examples including Adele, Pippa Middleton, Lorraine Pascale, the Food Network Chef and more

Instead of concentrating on ignoring a reader likes the food, the diet encourages increased consumption of such items such as wine, coffee and even dark chocolate. Inside all of us, these foods activate "sirtuin" genes; these genes regulate metabolism, stimulate weight loss and promote muscle growth. When Adele shares a picture of herself down 100 pounds on her 32nd birthday, it's a show stopper. We always marvel at the transformation of her body. We love and adore Adele at all sizes while you sit at home with your hand in chips, anything like that is always inspiring. Once Adele decided to slim down on her 2016/17 World Tour, she turned to trainer Pete Geracimo, who partnered with Goggins and Matten and had some of her clients on The Sirtfood Diet including Pippa Middleton, Kim Cattrall and UFC World Champion Conor McGregor. Four-time Olympic gold medalist Sir Ben Ainslie wrote, "Sirtfoods are important for me to hit new peaks in success to meet the challenges of making the history of British America's Cup."

Here is the diet that supposedly got Adele to her latest combat look is for all those who want to try it out. Or if you're going to lose 10 pounds, or like me, the 15 that I gained during this period of "working from home" (which I call working next to the refrigerator process), then try the Sirtfood diet.

By the way, the Sirtfood Diet has been adopted by many people, including Pippa Middleton, Lorraine Pascale, the Food Network Chef, the actress Jodi Kidd, Sir Ben Ainslie, and a boxer named David Haye. Sirt foods help signal your body to restore your metabolism and increase muscle mass while burning fat. The field of nutrition science was turned on its head when five-year research on more than 7,400 individuals found that specific diets reduced diabetes and heart disease by an astounding 30%. They avoided weight gain and stopped early death, all regardless of calorie, carbohydrate or fat consumption. Aidan Goggins and Glen Matten, specialists in nutritional medicine, studied a Sirtfood rich diet at their clinic in Britain's most prestigious private health club, KX, where guests include Adele, Daniel Craig, Pippa Middleton, Madonna and many royals. Members experienced a fast 7- pound fat loss in 7 days, held it off, and recorded well-being and energy bursts. Pete Geracimo, the celebrity trainer, whose clients include Adele and Pippa Middleton, suggests THE SIRTFOOD DIET as their hidden weapon. Geracimo addresses the demand of his customers for fulfilling food in his persuasive foreword, which fuels a jet-setter lifestyle, gets and keeps them at a healthy weight and ensures vibrant health and energy. Pete Geracimo, long-term and on tour trainer of Adele, says that he has put all his customers on The Sirtfood Diet and everybody looks great now – no deprivation necessary. The most famous argument is that it can motivate you to lose up to seven pounds a week, one of its founders Matten told. Adele's transformation also shows it over the years. But this isn't a cake: For three days just 1000 calories a day are eaten by eaters— one meal filled with sirtuins and two green juices. In the next four days, an additional meal will allow up to 1.500 calories to be bumped. After that week, you can eat as much sirt food as you want. Daily exercise on a diet is also advisable.

The foods should increase muscle growth because their "skin gene" activate the effects of diet and exercise. The foods are supposed to increase muscle growth.

A nutritionist, Martha McKittrick from Manhattan, said recently that the diet she believes is "skizzy." "Not everyone will be able to see the results from Adele," said Grace Fjeldberg, a registered dietitian.

However, this diet has been classified as the most searched 2019 diet for Google, "No. 7." according to Trudy Thelander, a co-creator of the Mediterranean diet — the original inspiration for the Sirt diet is scientifically sound.

German scientific study of the benefits of a Mediterranean diet that combines two of the world's healthiest diets— the Mediterranean and Asian,' she said. "The term 'Sirtfood' has come to be coined by German scientists from Kiel University."

Traditional Mediterranean and Asian diets are rich in compounds known as polyphenols of natural vegetables. The consumption by a special family of body genes called Sirtuins, which play an essential role in slowing down cell age, reducing inflammation and regulating blood sugars, of these polyphenolic foods — including extra virgin olive oil, peat, capers, green tea and red wines. The ability of the body to burn fat can be increased.

The researchers have found that the advantages of a Mediterranean diet which activates sirtuin are similar to severe calorie limiting (such as fasting) but without having to limit calories. The results have been obtained.

Their pioneering research was published in 2013. "We propose that a so-called "Mediterranean diet" combining sirtuin activated food (Sirtfood) from both the Asian and Mediterranean Diets may be a very promise-oriented dietary strategy for preventing chronic conditions, ensuring that people have healthy eating and good ageing." "Unlike modern, highly-processed Western diets, the Mediterranean foods rely on minimum-processed foods, such as vegetables, fruit, grains, boars, nuts, olive oil and fish. These foods are overflowing with health-promoting compounds, including omega-three fatty acids, plant chemicals, antioxidants and dietary fiber, which are good for good health and are also great for good health. "Eating this way is not at all restrictive, but it's very enjoyable," says Dietitian Caroline Fernandes. "Some of our best food is from Mediterranean and Asian regions such as Italy, Greece and

Japan. Patients are now recommending a Mediterranean diet, and the results were highly positive. "We observed, in practice, that patients don't feel in the limited sense of the word, in a diet but are transiting to a new way of life that implies the harmonious blend of flavors, food and seasonings."

Filled with encouraging case studies, easy-to-make recipes and a sustained performance maintenance plan, THE SIRTFOOD DIET tells you how you can lose 3 kg in seven days and hold it off while you build muscle. Take advantage of the power of the scientifically validated Sirtfood system from Goggins and Matten to enable weight loss, relieve aches and pains, sleep better, boost mood and alleviate cravings.

A Comparison of Typical and Sirtfood Diet Plan Typical Diet Plan

- Eat less, and work out more
- Interdict the food you want
- Slowing Metabolism
- Feeling hungry

- Lose muscle and strength
- Less power
- Temporary perks

Sirtfood Meal Plan

- Eat more, and work less
- Turn in to the food you enjoy
- Accelerate Metabolism
- Feel happy
- Develop strength and muscle
- Unlimited Energy
- Loss of weight and fitness for a whole life

2.2 Some Research about The Real Health Foods

More to Sirt than to body structure, too. More experimentally controlled trials on single Sirtfoods have shown good results outside of the Goggin's and Matten tests. For example, in October 2015, researchers at New York's Columbia University found that drinking water with a gram of cocoa – particularly rich in sirtuin activator epicatechin – dissolved therein led to improved memory in 19 middle-aged subjects.

Researchers at Monash University in Melbourne reported in November of the same year that, when patients in the type 2 diabetes early stages added one gram of turmeric a day to their diets, their working memory improved. There's some evidence for people with diabetes that sirtuin activation increases the amount of insulin that can be secreted and can make it function more efficiently. In the skeleton, the sirtuins encourage osteoblast growth and survival, a type of cell responsible for building new bone.

When more research is done, the next big thing for Sirt will be in its relation to leucine, the basic muscle-builder among the branched-chain amino acids.

Leucine is a crucial protein synthesis regulator and activates a protein known as mTOR (though you don't have to think about that to understand the next bit).

"Leucine is a double edge sword," Goggins explains "it's an acceleration for muscle development, but if you don't have the internal machinery to manage it, the engine can burst." In principle, getting a more sirtfood-heavy diet might increase the amount of protein your body will assimilate effectively, placing the old advice "20-30 g a sitting" firmly into the past. All that, of course, needs more research. Thirty-seven people in one gym are not much of sample size, and other studies have been done on the effects of sirtuins on animals or human cells – neither are they guaranteed to demonstrate what is going on inside the body accurately. But for all the controversies of the diet's more extreme statements, following some variant of the Sirt Diet, it's hard to see what you stand to lose. Even if you set aside the calorie-restricted version of the plan and leap straight into "maintenance" mode, you will eat a large variety of foods defined as essential in the so-called Blue Zones, world areas like Sardinia and Okinawa where people lead longer, healthier lives. "I don't like the word diet, but it's lifestyle-like diet as opposed to any quick-fix intervention," Donald says. "It's about living right, in essence. And given the popularity of green juice drinks, the general concept is about adding balanced whole natural ingredients rather than 'superfood' deification." Or, to put it some other way: you're unlikely to become less nutritious by having more kale, almonds, walnuts, and red wine into your diet, even if you're not a UFC fighter or a supermodel.

2.3 What are Some Top Sirtfoods?

The diet combines sirt foods and calorie restriction, which can both trigger the body to produce higher sirtuin levels.

- Kale
- Red wine
- Strawberries
- Onions
- Soy
- Parsley
- Extra virgin olive oil
- Dark chocolate (85% cocoa)
- Matcha green tea
- Buckwheat
- Turmeric
- Walnuts
- Arugula (rocket)
- Bird's eye chili
- Lovage
- Medjool dates
- Red chicory
- Blueberries
- Capers
- Coffee

2.4 What are the Phases of Sirtfood Diet

Lots of foods contain nutrients that cause sirtuin, but some include more than others. The writers of the diet mention the 20 best sirtfoods in their book 'The Sirtfood Diet' are: birds-eye chilies, buckwheat, capers, celery, chocolate, coffee, extra virgin olive oil, green tea, kale, lovage, Medjool dates, parsley, red chicory, red wine, rocket, rice, almonds, walnuts and turmeric.

Phases of Sirtfood Diet Plan

The diet is broken down into 2 phases.

Phase 1: The 'hyper success phase' of 7 days, incorporating a Sirtfood-rich diet with medium calorie restriction. Intake of calories is limited to 1,000 calories over the first three days (so, even more than on a five ratio two fasting day). The diet consists of 3 green juices rich in sirtfood and one meal rich in sirtfood and two squares of dark chocolate. Calories are increased to 1,500 calories over the remaining four days, and the diet includes two sirtfood-rich green juices and two sirtfood-rich meals each day. You are not permitted to drink any alcohol during Phase 1, but you are free to drink soda, tea, coffee and green tea.

Phase 2: The 'maintenance phase' of 14 days, where you maintain your weight loss without reducing calories.

We will discuss complete meal plan for your diet but let's go towards recipes and after that we will look how you have to follow these delicious recipes on daily basis. So, keep reading, there is everything you are looking for.

Chapter 3: Food List and Delicious Sirtfood Recipes

3.1 Foods to Buy When Following Sirtfood Diet

Before sirtfood meals and breakfast, you should have the following ingredients with you.

Drinks: Green tea (specifically Macha), coffee, Cocoa, Red wine.

Spices: Turmeric, Curry, Ginger, Chili, Cinnamon, Capers, Cloves, Cumin

Fruits: All dark berries, Apples, Dates, Lemons, Pomegranates

Vegetables: All leafy greens, Broccoli, Artichoke, Red onion, Celery,

Herbs: Parsley, Oregano, Peppermint, Rosemary, Thyme, Basil

Miscellaneous: Walnuts, Flax, Olives, Olive oil, Buckwheat, Soy, Chocolate

- **Bird's Eye Chilies:** They are sold as Thai chilies, more potent than traditional chilies, and more nutrient-packed as well. Utilize these to continue sweet and sour recipes.
- **Buckwheat:** Technically a pseudo-grain: it is a rhubarb-related fruit seed. It is also available in noodle form (as soba), but be sure to get the wheat-free version.
- **Capers:** They 're pickled flower buds in the event you 're curious. Sprinkle over lettuce or cauliflower toast.
- **Celery:** The most nutritious part is the hearts and leaves, so do not throw them away if you blend up a shake.
- **Cocoa:** The kind rich in flavonol improves blood pressure, regulation of blood sugar and cholesterol. Look for a large portion of cacao.
- Drink it dark-there is some evidence that milk can reduce sirtuin-activating nutrient absorption.

- **Extra Virgin Olive Oil:** The sort of extra virgin has more Sirt advantages, and a more pleasing, peppery taste.
- **Green Tea or Matcha:** Add one slice of lemon to improve sirtuin-producing nutrient absorption. Matcha is even better, but to prevent possible contamination with lead go to Japanese, not Chinese.
- **Kale:** Includes large amounts of quercetin and kaempferol, nutrients that activate sirtuin. Massage it with lemon juice and olive oil to serve as a salad.
- **Lovage:** It's more of an herb. On a windowsill, grow your own, and turn it into stir-fries.
- **Medjool Dates:** They are a heavy 66 percent sugar, but in moderation, they do not increase blood sugar levels and have been related to lower diabetes and heart disease rates.
- **Parsley:** It is more than just a garnish, in it Apigenin is high. To the full benefit, throw it into a smoothie or tea.
- **Chicory:** Red is great, but yellow does fit well. Put it out into a salad.
- **Red Onion:** For you, the red variety is better and good enough to eat raw. Chop it and add to a sandwich, or eat a burger with it.
- **Red Wine:** You've learnt about resveratrol: the good news is, it's heat resistant, so you can get advantages from cooking with it (as well as just glugging it). Pinot noir has the most quality.
- **Rocket Leaves:** It is from one of the least disturbed-with available green salads. Season with olive oil.
- **Soy:** Soybeans and miso are heavy on activators of sirtuin. Use these in stir-fries.
- **Strawberries:** While they are sweet, they contain just 1/100 g of sugar – and evidence indicates that they boost the capacity of your body to manage sugar carbs.
  - **Turmeric:** Data indicates that the curcumin has anti-cancer properties in it. Assimilating it alone is difficult for the body but boiling it in liquid and adding fat and

black pepper improves absorption.

- o **Walnuts:** These are High in calories and fat but well known to minimize metabolic disease. Smash them to a sirt-flavored pesto with parsley.

3.2 Sirtfood Diet Recipes for Breakfast

Recipe 1: Berry Soy Yogurt Parfait

This smooth berry soy yogurt parfait is one of my favorite, go-to breakfasts, snacks and even desserts. This Easy Berry Soy Yogurt Parfait is nutritious enough for a meal (rich in protein, carbohydrates, vitamins, minerals, phytochemicals), and delicious enough for a treat in which you can feel nice.

- Calories: 244
- Ready in: 2-4 minutes
- Servings: 1

Ingredients

- One 6-oz carton vanilla cultured soy yoghurt
- 1/4 cup granola (gluten-free)
- 1 cup berries (you can take strawberries, blueberries, raspberries, blackberries)

Instructions

- Put half of the yogurt in a glass jar or serving dish.
- On the top put half of the berries.
- Then sprinkle with half of granola
- Repeat layers.

Recipe 2: Sirt Muesli

Serves: 1

Ingredients

- 20g buckwheat flakes
- 10g buckwheat puffs
- 40g Medjool dates, pitted and chopped

- 15g walnuts, chopped
- 15g coconut flakes or desiccated coconut
- 100g strawberries, hulled and chopped
- 10g cocoa nibs
- 100g plain Greek yoghurt

Instructions

- You need to mix the dry ingredients and place them in an airtight container if you want to make it in a large amount or prepare it the night before. The next day all you need to do is add the strawberries and yoghurt, and it's good to go.

Recipe 3: Smoked Salmon Omelette

- Serves: 1

- Preparation Time: 5-10 minutes

- Calories: 288.1

Ingredients

- Medium eggs 2

- 100 g Smoked salmon, sliced

- 10 g Rocket, chopped

- 1/2 tsp Capers

- 1 tsp Parsley, chopped

- 1 tsp Extra virgin olive oil

Instructions

- Break the eggs in a bowl and stir well. Add the salmon, capers, parsley and rocket. In a non-stick frying pan, heat the olive oil until hot but not smoking. Add the egg mixture and move the mixture around the pan, using a spatula or fish slice, until it is even. Reduce fire, and let cook through the omelette. Stir spatula around the edges and roll the omelette up or fold in half to serve.

Recipe 4: Mushroom Scramble Egg

- Calories: 182
- Servings: 3
- Preparation Time: 5 minutes

Ingredients

- Two eggs
- 1 tsp ground turmeric
- 1 tsp mild curry powder
- 20g kale, roughly chopped
- 1 tsp extra virgin olive oil
- ½ bird's eye chili, thinly sliced
- a handful of thinly sliced, button mushrooms
- 5g parsley, finely chopped

Instructions

- Mix the curry and turmeric powder, then add a little water until a light paste has been achieved.
- Steam up the kale 2–3 minutes.
- At medium heat, heat the oil in a frying pan and fry the chili and mushrooms for 2–3 minutes till they start browning and softening.
- Put the eggs and spice paste, and cook over medium heat, then add the kale and start cooking for another minute over medium heat. Add the parsley, then mix well and serve.

Recipe 5: Matcha Green Tea Smoothie

This super-healthy smoothie makes use of matcha powder, a highly concentrated green Japanese tea. It can be found at Asian specialist or tea shops.

- Calories 183
- Preparation Time: 3 minutes
- Serves: 2

Ingredients

- 2 ripe bananas 2
- 2 tsp matcha green tea powder
- 2 tsp honey
- 1/2 tsp vanilla bean paste (not extract) or a small scrape of the seeds from a vanilla pod
- 250 ml of milk
- Six ice cubes

Instructions

- Blend all the ingredients in a blender and serve in two glasses.

Recipe 6: Date and Walnut Porridge

Now you start your day with this energetic porridge.

- Servings: 1
- Preparation Time: 10 minutes

Ingredients

- 200 ml Milk or dairy-free alternative
- 1 tsp. Walnut butter or four chopped walnut halves
- 1 Medjool date, chopped
- 50 g Strawberries, hulled
- 35 g Buckwheat flakes

Instructions

- Place the milk and date in a saucepan, heat gently, then add the buckwheat flakes and cook until the porridge is the consistency you like.
- Stir in the butter of walnut or walnuts, top with the strawberries and serve.

Recipe 7: Berry Chia Breakfast Bow

This naturally sweet, grain-free, gluten-free, sugar-free, vegan breakfast is a luscious way to start your day.

- Servings: 2
- Preparation Time: 10 minutes

Ingredients

- Eight pitted dates
- 1/2 cup canned coconut milk
- Two tablespoons blanched almonds or raw cashews
- Two teaspoons frozen orange juice concentrate
- One pinch salt
- 1/3 cup almond milk
- 1/2 teaspoon vanilla
- 2 cups diced, strawberries – divided
- 3/4 cup fresh blueberries
- 1/4 cup chia seed
- One small banana, sliced – optional

Instructions

- ✓ In a blender, place dates, coconut milk, almond milk, almonds, orange juice concentrate, cinnamon, salt, and 1 cup strawberries and mix until smooth.
- ✓ Shift mixture to medium bowl and stir in seed chia.
- ✓ Place in the fridge for a minimum of 2 hours, or overnight.
- ✓ Until serving, stir in the blueberries, remaining strawberries (sliced), and sliced bananas. Fresh berries work better than frozen.

Recipe 8: Green Omelette

- Calories: 234
- Ready in: 10 minutes
- Serves: 1

Ingredients

- 1 tsp olive oil
- Two large eggs, at room temperature
- 1 shallot, peeled and finely chopped
- Small handful (10g) parsley, finely chopped
- Handful (20g) rocket leaves
- Salt and freshly ground black pepper

Instructions

- In a frying pan heat, the oil at a medium to low heat and fry the shallot gently for 5 minutes. Switch the flame up a bit and then cook for another 2 minutes.

- Whisk the eggs well in a bowl or cup along with a fork. Distribute the shallot around the pan equally before pouring the eggs in m. Tip the pan slightly on either side to ensure an equal distribution of the egg. Cook for about a minute before you raise the sides of the omelette. Then allow any runny egg to slip into the base of the pan. Sprinkle leaves and parsley immediately over the shot, and season generously with salt and pepper.

- The top side of the omelette will still be soft but not runny when cooked, and the base will start browning. Spoon onto a plate and instantly enjoy.

3.3 Sirtfood Diet Salads and Lunch Recipes

Recipe 1: Turmeric Chicken and Kale Salad with Dressing of Honey Lime

Dress the salad 10 minutes before serving, if you cook it ahead of time. Chicken can be substituted with minced beef, chopped prawns or fish. Vegetarians may be using sliced mushrooms or cooked quinoa.

- Calories:
- Servings: 2
- Preparation Time: 20 minutes

Ingredients For Chicken

- 1 teaspoon of ghee or 1 tbsp. coconut oil
- 250–300 g / 9 oz. chicken mince or diced up chicken thighs
- 1teaspoon lime zest
- 1 teaspoon turmeric powder
- ½ medium brown onion, diced
- One large garlic clove, finely diced
- juice of ½ lime
- ½ teaspoon salt and pepper

For the salad

- Two tablespoons pumpkin seeds (pepitas)
- ½ avocado, sliced
- Three large kale leaves
- Broccolini stalks 6 or 2 cups of broccoli florets
- A handful of fresh parsley leaves, chopped
- A handful of fresh coriander leaves, chopped
- For the dressing
- Three tablespoons extra-virgin olive oil
- One teaspoon raw honey
- Three tablespoons lime juice
- ½ teaspoon wholegrain or Dijon mustard
- ½ teaspoon sea salt and pepper
- One small garlic clove, finely diced or grated

Instructions:

- In a small pan, warm the ghee or coconut oil over medium to high heat. Add the onion and sauté for 4-5 minutes on medium heat, until golden. Add the minced chicken and garlic and swirl over medium-high heat for 2-3 minutes, breaking it apart.

- Add the turmeric, lime zest, lime juice, salt and pepper and cook for a further 3-4 minutes, stirring frequently. Set aside the cooked slush.

- Make a small saucepan of water to boil while the chicken cooks. Stir in the broccolini and cook 2 minutes. Rinse under cold water, and cut into three or four bits each.

- Add the pumpkin seeds from the chicken into the frying pan and toast for 2 minutes at medium heat, whisking regularly to avoid burning. Season with a touch of salt. Keep it aside. Raw pumpkin seeds should also be used well.

- In a salad bowl, put the chopped kale, and pour over the dressing. Toss the kale with the dressing, and massage it with your palms. It will soften the kale, sort of like what citrus juice does to carpaccio fish or beef – it 'cooks' it a little bit.

- The cooked rice, broccolini, fresh herbs, pumpkin seeds and slices of avocado are eventually tossed.

Recipe 2: Miso Marinated Baked Cod

- Serves: 2

Ingredients

- 20g miso

- 1tbsp mirin

- 1tbsp extra virgin olive oil

- 200g skinless cod fillet

- 20g red onion, sliced

- One clove garlic, finely chopped

- 40g celery, sliced

- 1tsp fresh ginger, finely chopped

- One bird's eye chili, finely chopped

- 60g green beans

- 30g buckwheat

- 50g kale, roughly chopped

- 1tsp ground turmeric

- 5g parsley, roughly chopped

- 1tbsp tamari or soy sauce

- 1tsp sesame seeds

Instructions

- Heat the oven to 220 ° C/200oC a fan/gas limit of 7.

- Blend the miso, mirin and 1tsp oil, whisk in the cod and marinate 30 minutes. Transfer to a baking tray, then cook 10 minutes.

- Meanwhile, heat the remaining oil over a large frying pan. For a few minutes, add the onion and stir-fry, then add the celery, garlic, chili, ginger, green beans and kale. Keep frying until the kale is tender and cooked through, adding a little water if necessary to soften the kale.

- Cook the buckwheat with the turmeric as directed on the box. Attach the parsley, sesame seeds and tamari or soy sauce.

- Serve to the stir-fry with greens and fish.

Recipe 3: Baked Salmon Salad with Creamy Mint Dressing

- Calories: 340
- Servings: 1
- Time: 20 minutes

Ingredients

- One salmon fillet (130g)
- 40g mixed salad leaves

- Two radishes, trimmed and thinly sliced
- 40g young spinach leaves
- 5cm piece (50g) cucumber, cut into chunks
- One small handful (10g) parsley, roughly chopped
- Two spring onions, trimmed and sliced

For the dressing:

- 1 tbsp. natural yoghurt
- 1 tsp low-fat mayonnaise
- Two leaves mint, finely chopped
- 1 tbsp. rice vinegar
- Salt and freshly ground black pepper

Instructions:

- Firstly, you heat the oven to 200 ° C (180 ° C fan / Gas 6).
- Place the salmon filet on a baking tray and bake for 16–18 minutes until you have just cooked. Remove, and set aside from the oven. The salmon in the salad is equally nice and hot or cold. If your salmon has skin, cook the skin side down and remove the salmon from the skin after cooking, use a slice of fish. When cooked, it should slide away easily.
- Mix the mayonnaise, yoghurt, rice wine vinegar, mint leaves and salt and pepper in a small dish and let it to stand for at least 5 minutes for aromas to evolve.
- Place on a serving plate the salad leaves and spinach, and top with the radishes, the cucumber, the spring onions and the parsley. Flake the cooked salmon over the salad and sprinkle over the dressing.

Recipe 4: Lamb, Butternut Squash and Date Tagine

The lamb and onion 's natural juices produce steam which bastes the meat as it cooks over low flame. The gentle heat keeps the inside of the tagine moist and does not dry out or burn.

- Calories: 404

- Servings: 4 to 6
- Preparation Time: 15 minutes

Ingredients

- Two tablespoons olive oil
- 2cm ginger, grated
- One red onion, sliced
- Three garlic cloves, grated or crushed
- One teaspoon chili flakes (or to taste)
- One cinnamon stick
- Two teaspoons cumin seeds
- Two teaspoons ground turmeric
- ½ teaspoon salt
- 800g lamb neck fillet, cut into 2cm chunks

- 100g medjool dates, pitted and chopped
- 400g tin chopped tomatoes, plus half a can of water
- 400g tin chickpeas, drained
- 500g butternut squash, cut into 1cm cubes
- Two tablespoons fresh coriander (plus extra for garnish)
- Buckwheat, couscous, flatbreads or rice to serve

Instructions:

- Preheat the oven until 140C.
- Sprinkle about two tablespoons of olive oil in a large oven-proof casserole dish or cast iron pot. Put the sliced onion and cook on a gentle heat until the onions softened but not brown, with the lid on for about 5 minutes.
- Add chili, cumin, cinnamon and turmeric to the grated garlic and ginger. Remove well, and cook the lid off for one more minute. If it gets too dry, add a drop of water.
- Next, add pieces of lamb. In the onions and spices, stir well to coat the meat and then add salt, chopped dates and tomatoes, plus about half a can of water (100- 200ml).
- Bring the tagine to the boil, then put the lid on and put it for 1 hour and 15 minutes in your preheated oven.
- Add the chopped butternut squash and drained

chickpeas thirty minutes before the end of the cooking time. Stir all together, bring the lid back on and go back to the oven for the remaining 30 minutes of cooking.

- Remove from the oven when the tagine is finished, and stir through the chopped coriander. Serve with couscous, buckwheat, flatbreads, or basmati rice.
- Notes:
- If you don't own an oven-proof casserole dish or cast-iron casserole, cook the tagine in a regular casserole until it has to go into the oven and then transfer the tagine to a regular lidded casserole dish before placing it in the oven. Add 5 minutes of cooking time to provide enough time to heat the casserole dish.

Recipe 5: Fragrant Asian Hotpot

- Calories: 185
- Servings: 2
- Total time: 15 minutes

Ingredients

- 1 tsp tomato purée
- 1-star anise, crushed (or 1/4 tsp ground anise)
- Small handful (10g) parsley, stalks finely chopped
- Juice of 1/2 lime
- Small handful (10g) coriander, stalks finely chopped
- 500ml chicken stock, fresh or made with one cube
- 1/2 carrot, peeled and cut
- 50g beansprouts
- 50g broccoli, cut into small florets
- 1 tbsp. good-quality miso paste
- 100g raw tiger prawns
- 50g rice noodles that are cooked according to packet instructions
- 50g cooked water chestnuts, drained
- 100g firm tofu, chopped
- 20g sushi ginger, chopped

Instructions:

- In a large saucepan, put the tomato purée, star anise, parsley stalks, coriander stalks, lime juice and chicken stock and bring to boil for 10 minutes.
- Stir in the carrot, broccoli, prawns, tofu, noodles and water chestnuts and cook gently until the prawns are cooked. Take it from heat and stir in the ginger sushi and the paste miso.
- Serve sprinkled with peregrine leaves and coriander.

Recipe 6: Asian King Prawn Stir Fry with Buckwheat Noodles

- Servings: 1
- Preparation Time: 10 minutes

Ingredients

- 150g of shelled raw king prawns, deveined
- 2 tsp tamari
- 75g soba (buckwheat noodles)
- 2 tsp extra virgin olive oil
- One garlic clove, finely chopped
- One bird's eye chili, finely chopped
- 1 tsp finely chopped fresh ginger
- 40g celery, trimmed and sliced
- 20g red onions, sliced
- 75g green beans, chopped
- 50g kale, roughly chopped
- 5g lovage or celery leaves
- 100ml chicken stock

Instructions:

- Heat a frying pan over a high flame, then cook the prawns for 2–3 minutes in 1 teaspoon tamari and one teaspoon oil. Place the prawns onto a tray. Wipe the pan out with paper from the kitchen, as you will be using it again.
- Cook the noodles 5–8 minutes in boiling water, or as

directed on the packet. Drain and put away.

- Meanwhile, over medium-high heat, fry the garlic, chili and ginger, red onion, celery, beans and kale in the remaining oil for 2–3 minutes. Add the stock and boil, then cook for one or two minutes until the vegetables are cooked but crunchy.
- Add the prawns, noodles and leaves of lovage/celery to the pan, bring back to the boil, then remove and eat.

Recipe 7: Prawn Arrabbiata

- Serves: 1
- Preparation Time: 35 to 40 minutes

Ingredients

- 125-150 g Raw or cooked prawns (Ideally king prawns)
- 65 g Buckwheat pasta
- 1 tbsp. Extra virgin olive oil
- For arrabbiata sauce
- 40 g Red onion, finely chopped
- 1 Garlic clove, finely chopped
- 30 g Celery, finely chopped
- 1 Bird's eye chili, finely chopped
- 1 tsp Dried mixed herbs
- 1 tsp Extra virgin olive oil
- 2 tbsp. White wine (optional)
- 400 g Tinned chopped tomatoes
- 1 tbsp. Chopped parsley

Instructions

- Firstly, you fry the onion, garlic, celery and chili over medium-low heat and dry herbs in the oil for 1–2 minutes. Switch the flame to medium, then add the wine and cook 1 minute. Add the tomatoes and leave the sauce to cook for 20-30 minutes over medium-low heat until it has a nice rich consistency. If you feel the sauce becomes too thick, add some water.

- While the sauce is cooking, boil a pan of water, and cook the pasta as directed by the packet. Drain, toss with the olive oil when cooked to your liking, and keep in the pan until needed.
- Add the raw prawns to the sauce and cook for another 3–4 minutes until they have turned pink and opaque, then attach the parsley and serve. If you use cooked prawns add the parsley, bring the sauce to the boil and eat.
- Add the cooked pasta to the sauce, blend well, then serve gently.

Recipe 8: Turmeric Baked Salmon

- Servings: 1
- Preparation Time: 10-15 minutes

Ingredients

- 125-150 g Skinned Salmon
- 1 tsp ground turmeric
- 1 tsp Extra virgin olive oil
- 1/4 Juice of a lemon

For the spicy celery
- 40 g Red onion, finely chopped
- 1 tsp Extra virgin olive oil
- 60 g Tinned green lentils
- 1 cm fresh ginger, finely chopped
- 1 Garlic clove, finely chopped
- 1 Bird's eye chili, finely chopped
- 150 g Celery, cut into 2cm lengths
- 130 g Tomato, cut into eight wedges
- 1 tsp Mild curry powder
- 1 tbsp. Chopped parsley
- 100 ml Chicken or vegetable stock

Instructions

- Heat the oven to a six mark 200C / gas.
- Start with the dazzling celery. Heat over medium-low

heat a frying pan, add olive oil, then onion, garlic, ginger, chili and celery. Then you fry gently for 2–3 minutes or till softened but not colored, then put the curry powder and cook for another minute.

- Put the tomatoes, stock and lentils, then gently simmer for 10 minutes.
- Accordingly, how crunchy you like your celery you might want to increase or decrease the cooking time.
- Meanwhile, combine the turmeric, lemon juice and oil and rub over the salmon.
- Put on a baking tray and cook 8–10 minutes.
- Stir the parsley in the celery to finish, and serve with salmon.

Recipe 9: Greek Salad Skewers

- Two wooden skewers, soaked in water for 30 minutes before use
- Eight large black olives
- Eight cherry tomatoes
- One yellow pepper, cut into eight squares
- ½ red onion, chopped in half and separated into eight pieces
- 100g (about 10cm) cucumber, cut into four slices and halved
- 100g feta, cut into eight cubes

- **For the dressing:**
- 1 tbsp. extra virgin olive oil
- 1 tsp balsamic vinegar
- Juice of ½ lemon
- Few leaves basil, finely chopped (or ½ tsp dried mixed herbs to replace basil and oregano)
- A right amount of salt and freshly ground black pepper
- Few leaves oregano, finely chopped
- ½ clove garlic, peeled and crushed

Instructions

- Thread each skewer in the order with salad ingredients: olive, tomato, yellow pepper, red onion, cucumber, feta, basil, olive, yellow pepper, red ointment, cucumber, feta.
- Put all the ingredients of the dressing in a small bowl and blend well together. Pour over the spoils.

Recipe 10: Strawberry Tabbouleh

It is quick and easy to make in no time.

- Servings: 5

Ingredients

- 50g buckwheat
- 1tbsp ground turmeric
- 65g tomato
- 20g red onion
- 25g Medjool dates pitted
- 1tbsp capers
- 100g strawberries, hulled
- 30g parsley
- 1tbsp extra virgin olive oil
- 30g rocket
- Juice 1/2 lemon
- 80g avocado

Instructions

- Firstly, cook the buckwheat with the turmeric as directed on the pack. Drain, and keep cool.
- Cut the avocado, tomato, red onion, dates, capers and parsley to taste and mix with the cooled buckwheat.
- Slice the strawberries and mix the oil and lemon juice gently in the salad on the rocket serve.

Recipe 11: Sesame Chicken Salad

- Calories: 304
- Servings: 2

- Ready in 12 minutes

Ingredients

- 1 tbsp. Mushroom

- sesame seeds

- 100g baby kale, roughly chopped

- One cucumber, peeled, halved lengthways, deseeded with a teaspoon and sliced

- ½ red onion, very finely sliced

- 60g pak choi, very finely shredded

- 150g cooked chicken, shredded

- Large handful (20g) parsley, chopped

For the dressing

- 1 tbsp. extra virgin olive oil

- 1 tsp clear honey

- Juice of 1 lime

- 2 tsp soy sauce

- 1 tsp sesame oil

Instructions

- Roast the sesame seeds for 2 minutes in a dry frying pan, until slightly brown and fragrant. Transfer to cool plate.

- Mix the olive oil, sesame oil, lime juice, honey and soy sauce in a small bowl to form a dressing.

- Put the cucumber, kale, pak choi, red onion and parsley in a large bowl and combine gently. Pour over the sauce, then again blend.

- Spread the salad with the grilled chicken between two plates, and top. Just before eating, brush over the sesame seeds.

Recipe 12: Creamy Kale and Stilton Soup

It is a tasty and straightforward Kale Soup. Enjoy it on a rainy evening to entertain yourself.

- Preparation Time: 10 minutes
- Servings: 4

Ingredients

- One large potato
- 200g chopped kale
- 1-litre vegetable stock
- 3 tbsp. double cream
- Fresh nutmeg
- 100g Stilton Cheese

Instructions

- In a large saucepan, placed one big peeled and diced potato and 1 liter of hot stock. Give lid, and bring to the boil and cook until potato is tender for 10 mints.
- Add 200 g of chopped kale and 100 g of Stilton crumbled, cover, and cook for another 5 minutes.
- Add 3 tbsp. of double milk, and a generous fresh nutmeg grating. Season well, then mix half of the soup before stirring back into the unblended half.
- Serve with some extra Crumbled Stilton on top.

Recipe 13: Sirt Fruit Salad Nutritional fact

- Calories: 186
- 3 of your SIRT 5 a day
- This fruit salad is full of the best fruit containing SIRTs.
- Serves 1:
- Cooking time:
- Ready in 10 minutes

Ingredients

- ½ cup freshly made green tea
- 1 tsp honey

- one orange halved
- 1 apple, cored and roughly chopped
- 10 red seedless grapes
- 10 blueberries

Instructions

- Stir in half a cup of green tea with the sugar. Once its dissolved, add half the orange juice. Put on to cool down.
- Cut the other half of the orange and place the chopped apple, grapes, and blueberries together in a bowl. Put it over the cooled tea, and leave to steep before serving for a few minutes.

Recipe 13: Fresh Saag Paneer

- Nutrition Fact: consists of 279 calories

- 3 of your SIRT 5 a day

- **Serves 2**

- cooking time: Ready in 20 minutes

Ingredients

- 2 tsp rapeseed oil

- 200g paneer. cut into cubes

- Salt and freshly ground black pepper

- One red onion, chopped

- One small thumb (3 cm) fresh ginger, peeled and cut into matchsticks

- One clove garlic, peeled and thinly sliced

- One green chili, deseeded and finely sliced

- 100g cherry tomatoes halved

- 1/2 tsp ground coriander

- 1/2 tsp ground cumin

- 1/4 tsp ground turmeric

- 1/2 tsp mild chili powder

- 1/2 tsp salt

- 100g fresh spinach leaves

- Small handful (10g) parsley, chopped

- Small handful (10g) coriander, chopped

Instructions

- Heat oil in a wide frying pan with lid. Keep the heat high.

- Now season the paneer generously with salt and pepper and toss into the pan. Fry for a few minutes until it becomes golden. Remove from the pan and set it aside.

- Reduce the heat and add the onion. Then fry for 5 minutes before adding the chili, garlic and ginger. Cook for a few more minutes before adding the cherry tomatoes. Give the lid on the saucepan and cook for another five minutes.

- Add the salt and spices then stir. Give the paneer back to the pan and stir until coated. Attach the spinach with the parsley and coriander to the saucepan and place on the lid.

- Allow 1-2 minutes for the spinach to wilt.

- Then put in the dish. Serve straight away.

3.4 Sirtfood Diet Dinner Recipes

Recipe 1: Baked Potatoes with Spicy Chickpea

This Spicy Chickpea Stew is delicious and makes a perfect topping for baked potatoes, plus it just happens to be vegetarian, organic, gluten-free and milk-free. And it has chocolate in it. It is a basic vegan dish, and it will warm up those cold winter nights.

- Calories 243
- Servings: 4-6
- Preparation Time: 10 minutes

Ingredients

- 4-6 baking potatoes, pricked all over
- Two tablespoons olive oil
- Two red onions, finely chopped
- Four cloves garlic, grated or crushed
- 2cm ginger, grated
- Two tablespoons turmeric
- ½ -2 teaspoons of chili flakes (depending on how hot you like things)
- Two tablespoons cumin seeds
- Splash of water
- Two into 400g tins chopped tomatoes
- Two tablespoons unsweetened cocoa powder (or cacao)
- Two into 400g tins chickpeas (or kidney beans if you prefer) including the chickpea water
- Two yellow peppers (or whatever color you prefer!), chopped into bite size pieces
- Two tablespoons parsley plus extra for garnish
- Salt and pepper to taste (optional)
- Side salad (optional)

Instructions

- Preheat the oven to 200C so you can make all the ingredients you need.
- Put your baking potatoes in the oven when the oven is hot enough, and cook them for an hour or till they are cooked as you want them.
- Put the olive oil and chopped red onion in a big broad saucepan once the potatoes are in the oven and cook gently with the lid until the onions are soft but not brown for 5 minutes.
- Remove the lid and add the garlic, cumin, ginger and

chili. Cook on low heat for another minute, then you add the turmeric and a tiny sprinkle of water and cook for another minute, keeping in mind not to let the saucepan get too dry.

- Add cocoa (or cacao) powder, chickpeas (including chickpea water) and yellow pepper in the tomatoes. Boil it and simmer for 45 minutes at low heat until the sauce is thick and greasy (but don't let it burn!). Stew will be handled roughly at the same time as the potatoes.
- At last, mix in the two tablespoons of parsley and some salt and pepper, if desired, and serve the stew over the baked potatoes, maybe with a small side salad.

Recipe 2: Coronation Chicken Salad

It is ready in a flash, and also safe. Put back those menus you took from where you found them!

- Calories: 289
- Servings: 2
- Preparation Time: 5 minutes

Ingredients

- Two skinless chicken breasts
- 3 tbsp. olive oil
- 2 tbsp. mango chutney (we like Bay Tree)
- 1/2 lemon
- 2 tbsp. toasted flaked almond
- 1/2 cucumber, sliced into sticks
- 50g bag watercress
- 1 tsp mild or medium curry powder

Instructions

- Toss the chicken breasts along with the curry powder and 1 tbsp. of oil. Heat a large non-stick pan and cook the chicken on each side for 5-6 mints until it is golden and cooked, then cut into strips.
- With a firm squeeze of lemon juice, whisk the remaining

oil and mango chutney together. Then, toss the cucumber, watercress, chicken and most of the flaked almonds in a large bowl. Divide it between two cups, scatter with the rest of the almonds and enjoy some on the side of the crusty bread.

Recipe 3: Kale and Red Onion Dhal with Buckwheat

The Kale and red onion dhal with buckwheat is delicious and very nutritious, quick and easy to make and naturally gluten-free, dairy-free, vegetarian and vegan.

- Preparation Time: 5 minutes
- Servings: 4

Ingredients

- One tablespoon olive oil
- One small red onion, sliced
- Three garlic cloves, grated or crushed
- One bird eye chili, deseeded and finely chopped (more if you like things hot!)
- 2 cm ginger, grated
- Two teaspoons turmeric
- Two teaspoons garam masala
- 160g red lentils
- 200ml water
- 400ml coconut milk
- 160g buckwheat (or brown rice)
- 100g kale

Instructions

- In a big, deep saucepan, put the olive oil and add the sliced onion. Cook at low pressure, with the lid on until softened for 5 minutes.
- Add the garlic, chili and ginger and cook for 1 minute.
- Add the turmeric, garam masala, sprinkle with water and cook for 1 minute.
- Add the red lentils, coconut milk and 200 ml of water (fill

the coconut milk with water and drop it into the casserole).

- Thoroughly mix everything and cook over a gentle heat for 20 minutes with the lid on. If the dhal starts sticking, stir periodically and add a little more water.
- After 20 minutes, add the Kale, whisk thoroughly and remove the lid and cook for another 5 minutes (1-2 minutes if spinach is used instead!)
- Place the buckwheat in a medium saucepan about 15 minutes before the curry is ready, and put plenty of boiling water. Bring the water again to the boil and cook for 10 minutes (or much longer if you prefer softer buckwheat. Pour the buckwheat in a sieve and serve with the dhal.

Recipe 4: Aromatic Chicken

- Servings: 1
- Preparation Time: 15 minutes

Ingredients

For the salsa

- One large tomato
- One bird's eye chili, finely chopped
- 1tbsp capers, finely chopped
- 5g parsley, finely chopped
- Juice 1/2 lemon

For the chicken
- 120g skinless, boneless chicken breast
- 2tsp ground turmeric
- Juice 1/2 lemon
- 1tbsp extra virgin olive oil
- 50g kale, chopped
- 20g red onion, sliced
- 1tsp fresh ginger, finely chopped
- 50g buckwheat

Instructions

- Heat the oven at 220oC/200oC fan/gas level 7
- Cut the tomato thinly to make the salsa and make sure you hold as much of the liquid as possible. Mix with the chili, capers, lemon juice and parsley.
- Marinate the chicken breast for 5-10 minutes with 1tsp of turmeric, lemon juice and half of the butter.
- Heat the frying pan ovenproof, add the marinated chicken and cook each side for a minute until golden, then move to the oven for 8-10 minutes or until cooked through. Remove and cover with tape, then leave for 5 minutes to rest.
- Then you cook the Kale in a 5-minute steamer. In the remaining oil, fry the onion and ginger until soft but not white, then put the cooked Kale and fry for one more minute.
- Cook the buckwheat with the remaining turmeric as directed, then serve.

Recipe 5: Chargrilled Beef with a Red wine jus, Onion rings, Garlic kale and Herb roasted Potatoes

Steak strips on a bed of steamed garlic kale, sliced red onion and crispy herb-roasted potatoes are perfectly prepared.

- Servings: 1
- Total Time: 50 minutes

Ingredients

- 100g potatoes, peeled and cut into dice of 2cm
- 5g parsley, finely chopped
- 1 tbsp. extra virgin olive oil
- 50g kale, sliced
- 50g red onion, sliced into rings
- One garlic clove, finely chopped
- 150ml beef stock
- 120–150g into a 3.5cm-thick beef fillet steak
- 40ml red wine

- 1 tsp of tomato puree
- 1 tsp corn flour, dissolved in 1 tbsp. of water

Instructions

- The oven heats up to 220oC / gas 7.
- Place the potatoes in a boiling water saucepan, bring them back to boil and cook for 4–5 minutes, then drain. Put one teaspoon of oil in a roasting pan, and roast for 35–45 minutes in the hot oven. Switch the potatoes every 10 minutes to ensure cooking is all finished. Remove from the oven when cooked, sprinkle with the chopped parsley and stir well.

- Fry the onion for 5–7 minutes over medium heat in 1 teaspoon of butter, until soft and beautifully caramelized. Hold on warm. Steam the kale then drain for 2–3 minutes. Gently fry the garlic in 1/2 teaspoon of oil for 1 minute, until it is soft but not colored. Attach the kale and fry, until tender, for a further 1–2 minutes. Hold on warm.
- Heat a frying pan which is ovenproof over high heat until it is smoking. Coat the meat in 1/2 teaspoon of oil and fry over medium-high heat in the hot pan, depending on how you like your meat cooked. If you prefer your meat medium, it will be easier to sear the meat and then move the pan to a 220oC / gas seven oven and finish the cooking according to the specified times.
- Remove the meat from the saucepan and put to rest. To pick up any meat odor add the wine to the hot pan. Bubble to halve the juice, with a concentrated flavor, before syrupy.
- Add the puree of the stock and tomato to the steak pan and bring to boil, then add the corn flour paste to thicken the sauce, apply it a little at a time until the perfect consistency has been achieved. Add some of the remained steak juices and serve with the roasted potatoes, kale, onion rings and red wine sauce.

Recipe 6: Buckwheat Noodles with Chicken kale & Miso Dressing

Look 100 percent buckwheat noodles in Asian grocery stores to appreciate the delicious nutty flavor of buckwheat. A little spiciness is required in the light, gingery dressing, so use a good pinch of cayenne or other hot pepper. This version is supposed to be a little first-course salad.

- Calories: 253
- Servings: 2
- Preparation Time: 15 minutes

Ingredients

For the noodles

- 2-3 handfuls of kale leaves (removed from the stem and roughly cut)

- 3-4 shiitake mushrooms, sliced

- 150 g / 5 oz. buckwheat noodles (100% buckwheat, no wheat)

- One teaspoon coconut oil or ghee

- One medium free-range chicken breast, sliced or diced

- One brown onion, finely diced

- One long red chili, thinly sliced (seeds in or out depending on how hot you like it)

- Two large garlic cloves, finely diced

- 2-3 tablespoons Tamari sauce (gluten-free soy sauce)

For the miso dressing

- One tablespoon Tamari sauce

- 1½ tablespoon fresh organic miso

- One tablespoon extra-virgin olive oil

- One teaspoon sesame oil (optional)

- One tablespoon lemon or lime juice

Instructions

- Bring a medium water saucepan to boil. Add the kale and cook until slightly withered, for 1 minute. Remove and set aside, then put the water back to the boil. Add the soba noodles and cook (usually about 5 minutes) according to packaging instructions. Set aside and rinse under cold water.

- Meanwhile, in a little ghee or coconut oil (about a teaspoon), pan fry the shiitake mushrooms for 2-3 minutes, until lightly browned on either side. Sprinkle with salt from the sea, and set aside.

- Heat more coconut oil or ghee in the same frying pan over medium to high heat. Stir in onion and chili for 2-3 minutes, then add pieces of chicken. Cook over medium heat for 5 minutes, stirring a few times, then add the garlic, tamari sauce and some splash of water. Cook for another 2-3 minutes, often stirring until chicken is cooked through.

- Finally, add the kale and soba noodles and warm up by stirring through the chicken.

- In the end, mix the miso dressing and drizzle over the noodles to keep all the beneficial probiotics alive and active in the miso.

Recipe 8: Sirt Super Salad Serving: 1
Ingredients

- 50g rocket
- 50g chicory leaves
- 100g smoked salmon slices
- 80g avocado, peeled, stoned and sliced
- 40g celery, sliced
- 20g red onion, sliced
- 15g walnuts, chopped

- One large Medjool date, pitted and chopped
- 1tbsp extra virgin olive oil
- 1tbsp capers
- Juice 1/2 lemon
- 10g parsley, chopped
- 10g lovage or celery leaves, chopped

Instructions

- Mix all the ingredients, and your salad is ready.

Recipe 9: Baked Chicken Breasts

Ready in: 30 minutes

For the pesto

- 15g parsley
- 15g walnuts
- 15g Parmesan
- 1tbsp extra virgin olive oil
- Juice 1/2 lemon

For the chicken

- 150g skinless chicken breast
- 20g red onions, finely sliced
- 1tsp red wine vinegar
- 35g rocket
- 100g cherry tomatoes halved
- 1tsp balsamic vinegar

Instructions

- Heat the oven 220 ° C/200oC to a fan/gas limit of 7.
- To make pesto, blend in a food processor the parsley, walnuts, parmesan, olive oil, half the lemon juice and 1 tbsp. of water until you have done
- Paste smooth. Gradually add more water until you get the consistency you prefer.
- In the refrigerator, marinate the chicken breast in 1 tbsp. of pesto and the remaining lemon juice for 30 minutes or

longer, if possible.

- Fry the chicken in its marinade for 1 minute on either side in an oven-proof frying pan over medium-high heat, then move to the oven and cook for 8 minutes, or until cooked through.
- Marinate the red wine vinegar with the onions for 5-10 minutes, then drain the liquid.
- Remove the chicken from the oven, spoon over 1 tbsp. of pesto and let the heat from the chicken melt. Make a cover with foil and leave for 5 minutes to rest before serving.
- Combine the balsamic with the rocket, tomatoes and onion and drizzle over it. Serve with the chicken and spoon the rest of the pesto.

Recipe 10: Kale, Edamame and Tofu Curry

- Calories: 342
- Read time: 45 minutes
- Servings: 4

Ingredients

- One large onion, chopped
- 1 tbsp. rapeseed oil
- One large thumb (7cm) fresh ginger, peeled and grated
- Four cloves garlic, peeled and grated
- One red chili, deseeded and thinly sliced
- 1/2 tsp ground turmeric
- 1/4 tsp cayenne pepper
- 1 tsp paprika
- 1 tsp salt
- 1/2 tsp ground cumin
- 250g dried red lentils
- 50g frozen soya edamame beans
- 1 liter boiling water
- Two tomatoes, roughly chopped
- 200g firm tofu, cut into cubes
- 200g kale leaves stalk removed and torn

- Juice of 1 lime

Instructions

- Place the oil over low-medium heat into a heavy-bottomed pan. Add the onion and cook for 5 minutes before adding the garlic, ginger and chili, then cook for another 2 minutes. Add the turmeric, cayenne, cumin, paprika and salt. Remove and stir again, before adding the red lentils.
- Pour in the boiling water and cook for 10 minutes until the curry has a thick 'porridge' consistency, then rising the heat and cook for another 20-30 minutes.
- Add the soya beans, tofu and tomatoes and start cooking for another 5 minutes. Add the juice of lime and kale leaves, and cook until the kale is tender.

Recipe 12: Lamb, Butternut Squash and Date Tagine

- Preparation time: 15 minutes
- Cooking time: 1 hour 15 minutes
- Total time: 1 hour 30 minutes

Note

- This recipe's incredible warming Moroccan spices make this healthy tagine perfect for chilly autumn. It is also suitable for winter evenings.
- You can serve with buckwheat for an extra health kick.

Serving

- Serves: 4

Ingredients

- Two tablespoons olive oil
- One red onion, sliced
- 2cm ginger, grated
- Three garlic cloves, grated or crushed
- One teaspoon chili flakes (or to taste)
- Two teaspoons cumin seeds
- One cinnamon stick

- Two teaspoons of ground turmeric
- 800g of lamb neck fillet that is cut into 2cm chunks
- 100g Medjool dates, pitted and chopped
- ½ teaspoon of salt
- 500g butternut squash, cut into 1cm cubes
- 400g tin chopped tomatoes, with half a can of water
- 400g tin chickpeas, drained
- Two tablespoons fresh coriander (plus extra
- for garnish)
- Buckwheat, couscous, flatbreads or rice to serve

Instructions

- Preheat your oven to 140C.
- Put about two tablespoons of olive oil into an ovenproof pan or cast iron casserole dish. Put the chopped onion and cook on a gentle heat, with the lid on, for about 5 minutes. You can do it till the onions get softened but not brown.
- Add the garlic and ginger, chili, cumin, cinnamon and turmeric. Stir well and cook for one more minute by taking off the lid. Put a splash of water if it becomes dry.
- Then, you put in the lamb chunks. Mix for covering the meat in the onions and spices and then put the salt, chopped dates and tomatoes, along with about half a can of water (100-200ml).
- Make the tagine to the boil. Then give the lid on and place in your heated oven for about 1 hour and 15 minutes.
- Put in the chopped butternut squash and drained chickpeas, thirty minutes before the end of the cooking time. Stir all the things together, give the lid back on. Then put it back to the oven for the last 30 minutes of cooking.
- When the tagine gets ready, take it out from the oven and mix with the chopped coriander. You can serve with buckwheat, flatbreads, couscous, or basmati rice.

Notes

- If you don't have an ovenproof saucepan or cast iron casserole dish, cook the tagine in a normal saucepan up till it is ready to go in the oven and then shift the tagine into a regular lid casserole dish before putting in the oven. Give an extra 5 minutes of cooking time to allow for the fact that the casserole dish will need additional time to heat up.)

Recipe 13: Tuscan Bean Stew Ingredients

- 1 tbsp. extra virgin olive oil

- 50g red onion, finely chopped

- 30g celery, trimmed and finely chopped

- One garlic clove, finely chopped

- 30g carrot, peeled and finely chopped

- ½ bird's eye chili, finely chopped (optional)

- 1 tsp herbs de Provence

- 200ml vegetable stock

- 40g buckwheat

- 1 x 400g tin chopped Italian tomatoes

- 1 tsp tomato purée

- 1 tbsp. roughly chopped parsley

- 50g kale, roughly chopped

- 200g tinned mixed beans

Instructions

- ✓ Put the oil over low to medium heat in a medium saucepan and fry the onion, carrot, celery, garlic, chili and herbs gently until the onion is soft but not colored.

- ✓ Stir in stock, tomatoes, and purée tomatoes and bring to boil. Add the beans and allow to cook for 30 minutes.

✓ Add the kale and cook for another 5–10 minutes, then add the parsley, until tender.

✓ In the meantime, cook the buckwheat as instructed by the packet, drain and then serve with stew.

3.5 Sirtfood Diet Smoothies and Drinks Recipes

Recipe 1: Kale and Blackcurrant Smoothie

It is a delicious recipe for blackcurrant smoothie. This non-alcoholic mixed drink is straightforward and tasty. Using some (fresh or frozen) berries for this recycle.

- Calories: 86
- Servings: 2
- Preparation Time: 2-4 minutes

Ingredients

- 2 tsp honey
- Ten baby kale leaves stalk removed
- One ripe banana
- Six ice cubes
- 1 cup freshly made green tea
- 40 g blackcurrants, washed and stalks removed

Instructions

- Drop the honey into the warm green tea until it dissolves. Whiz all of the ingredients in a blender together until smooth. Serve straight away.

Recipe 2: Grape and Melon Juice

- Calories: 125
- Servings: 1
- Preparation Time: 2 minutes

Ingredients

- ½ cucumber, peeled
- 30g stalks removed, young spinach leaves

- 100g red grapes seedless
- 100g of cantaloupe melon, peeled, deseeded

Instructions

- Mix all the ingredients in a juicer or blender until smooth.

Recipe 3: Green Juice

This green juice is packed with Sirtfoods rich in nutrients, perfect for anyone who wants a little health boost and essential for anyone following the Sirtfood Diet.

- Calories: 90
- Servings: 1
- Preparation Time: 5 minutes

Ingredients

- 30g rocket
- 75g kale
- Two celery sticks
- 5g parsley
- 1cm ginger
- ½ green apple
- Juice of ½ lemon
- ½ teaspoon matcha green tea

Instructions

- Juice all the ingredients except lemon and green matcha tea.
- Manually squeeze the lemon juice into the green juice.
- Pour a little green juice into a glass and whisk in the matcha. Put the remaining green juice into the bottle, then mix again.
- Drink immediately or save for later.

Recipe 4: Matcha Green Tea

It is considered as a super sirtfood and is considered as a key component of sirtfood diet.

- Calories: 20
- Preparation Time: 30 seconds

Ingredients

- 1 cup ice
- Two teaspoons matcha powder
- Chilled unsweetened vanilla almond milk 2-3 ounces
- 1/2 cup cold water
- Dash of vanilla or chai spice, or some fresh mint

Instructions

- Pour ice into a bottle, or shaker, and sift into a shaker two teaspoons of matcha powder. Apply half a cup of cold water, shake the mixture well and pour in an ice- filled bottle. (The tea doesn't boil or dissolve, mixes in. If you allow it to stay for a while after shaking, the tea can fall to the edge, so quickly stir it or shake it again to get it mixed in!) When we make this a latte, we put 2-3 ounces of cold, unsweetened vanilla almond milk into the glass and sometimes whisk in a splash of coffee or chai spice–or some fresh mint, depending on our mood!

Recipe 5: Sirt Wonder Smoothie Ingredients
- One handful of Arugula (Rocket)
- One handful of Kale
- 2 handfuls of organic Strawberries
- Juice of ½ an organic lemon or lime
- 175ml filtered water
- ½ handful of Watercress
- ½ a teaspoon of matcha green tea
- 3 sprigs of Parsley

Instructions

- Put all the ingredients to a blender except matcha, and whizz until really smooth. Add the green tea powder to the matcha and send it a final blast until well balanced.

3.6 Sirtfood Desserts

Recipe 1: Sirtfood Chocolate Bites

- Servings: It makes 15-20 bites
- Preparation Time: 5 minutes

Ingredients

- 120g walnuts
- 30g dark chocolate (85% cocoa solids), broken into pieces, or cocoa nibs
- 1tbsp cocoa powder
- 250g Medjool dates pitted
- 1tbsp extra virgin olive oil
- 1tbsp ground turmeric
- Scraped seeds of 1 vanilla pod

Instructions

- Put the walnuts and chocolate in a food processor and blend until a fine powder is in. Put all the other ingredients, and blend until a big ball shapes the mixture. Add 2tbsp water if appropriate, to help tie it.

Make bite-sized balls from the mixture with your hands and refrigerate for at least 1 hour before serving in an airtight dish. The balls can stay safe in the fridge for up to a week.

Recipe 2: Chocolate Cupcakes with Matcha Icing

- Serves:12

- Time: 35 minutes

- Calories: 234

Ingredients

- 200g caster sugar
- 150g self-rising flour
- 60g cocoa
- ½ tsp fine espresso coffee, decaf if preferred
- ½ tsp salt
- ½ tsp vanilla extract
- 120ml milk
- 50ml vegetable oil
- One egg
- 120ml boiling water

For the icing

- 50g butter, at room temperature
- 1 tbsp. matcha green tea powder
- ½ tsp vanilla bean paste
- 50g soft cream cheese
- 50g icing sugar

Instructions

- Preheat the fan from oven to 180C/160C. Line a paper or silicone cake case with cupcake tin.

- In a big bowl, put the flour, sugar, cocoa, salt and espresso powder and thoroughly mix in.

- In addition to the dry ingredients, add the milk, vanilla extract, vegetable oil and egg and take help of an electric mixer to beat until well combined. Pour in the boiling water carefully slowly and beat at low velocity until thoroughly combined. Using a high-velocity beat to add air to the batter for another minute. The batter is significantly more liquid than a regular cake mix. Have faith, and it'll taste incredible!

- Kindly spoon the batter between the cake cases. Per cake box should be no more than 3/4 complete. Bake for 15-18 minutes in the oven, until the mixture, bounces back when squeezed. Take out from the oven, and set to cool before icing completely.

- Cream the butter and icing the sugar until it is pale and smooth. Add the vanilla and matcha powder, and stir again. Add the cream cheese, then beat until smooth. Pip or sprinkle over the cakes.

Recipe 3: Raspberry and Blackcurrant Jelly-Sirtfood

Preparing a jelly beforehand is a perfect way to prepare the fruit, so it is ready to eat first thing in the morning.

- Calories: 76

- Serves: 2

- Preparation Time: 15 minutes

Ingredients

- Two leaves gelatin

- 100g raspberries washed

- 100g blackcurrants washed and stalks removed

- 2 tbsp. granulated sugar

- 300ml water

Instructions

- Assemble the raspberries in two dishes/glasses/molds to eat. Place the gelatin leaves softening in a bowl of cold water.

- Put the blackcurrants with the sugar and 100ml water in a small saucepan and bring to a boil. Simmer hard for 5 minutes, then remove from oil. Leave on for 2 minutes.

- Squeeze the gelatin leaves out of the excess water and return to the saucepan. Remove until fully dissolved, then mix in the remaining water. Pour the liquid into the prepared dishes and set aside to cool. The jellies should be ready overnight or in about 3-4 hours.

Recipe 4: Apple Pancakes with Blackcurrant Compote-Sirtfood

Those are decadent yet nutritious pancakes — a super lazy treat in the morning.

- Calories: 337
- Serves: 4
- Ready in 20 minutes

Ingredients

- 75g porridge oats

- 125g plain flour

- 1 tsp baking powder

- 2 tbsp. caster sugar

- Pinch of salt

- 300ml semi-skimmed milk

- Two apples, peeled, cored and cut

- Two egg whites

- 2 tsp light olive oil

For the compote:

- 120g blackcurrants washed and stalks removed

- 3 tbsp. water

- 2 tbsp. caster sugar

Instructions

- Make the compote, first. Put the blackcurrants, sugar and water in a small saucepan. Bring to a cooker and simmer for 10-15 minutes.

- In a big bowl, add the oats, flour, baking powder, caster sugar and salt and combine well. Stir in the apple and whisk a little at a time in the milk until you have a smooth blend. Whisk the egg whites to firm peaks, then fold into the batter for the pancake. Bring the batter over to a tub.

- Heat 1/2 tsp of oil over medium-high heat in a non- stick frying pan and pour approximately one-quarter of the batter. Cook until golden brown, on both sides. Remove for four pancakes and repeat to make.

- Serve the pancakes drizzled over with blackcurrant compote.

Recipe 5: Pineapple Buckwheat Pancake

Such pineapple buckwheat pancakes are speckled with new pineapple hemp seeds and whole rings. They 're the perfect balance between sweet and heartful.

- Calories: 316

- Servings: 4

- Preparation Time: 15 minutes

Ingredients

- 1 cup buckwheat flour

- 1/4 cup almond flour

- Two tablespoons hemp seeds, plus more for topping

- One teaspoon baking powder

- 1/2 teaspoon allspice

- 5.3 ounces' pineapple Muuna cottage cheese

- One egg

- One teaspoon vanilla extract

- 2 tablespoon of maple syrup, plus more for serving

- One tablespoon butter, divided

- 1 cup unsweetened almond milk

- One small pineapple, outer layer cut off, sliced into rings and cored, (you can also use canned pineapple rings)
- 1/4 teaspoon salt

Instructions

- Prepare a medium-heat pancake griddle or skillet.
- In a wide bowl, mix flours, hemp seeds, baking powder, allspice, and salt, and whisk until mixed.
- In the bowl, add the cottage cheese, egg, maple syrup, and vanilla. Whisk in as you add the milk gradually until all is well mixed.
- Add a bit of butter to the saucepan. Place one pineapple ring on top once melted, cook until golden brown and start caramelizing. Flip the slice of pineapple over, spoon pancake batter on top, so it fills the ring and spills a little over the edges. Cook until set (about 3 minutes), turn carefully on the other side and cook for another 2 minutes.
- Repeat with remaining batter and pineapple rings.
- Serve to top with maple syrup and extra hemp seeds.

Recipe 6: Choc Chip Granola Recipe

Breakfast with Chocolate! Be sure to serve with a cup of green tea to provide you with lots of SIRTs. If you prefer the rice malt syrup can be replaced with maple syrup.

- Calories: 244
- Serves: 8
- Time: 30 minutes

Ingredients:

- 200g jumbo oats
- 50g pecans, roughly

- chopped
- 3 tbsp. light olive oil
- 20g butter
- 1 tbsp. dark brown sugar
- 2 tbsp. rice malt syrup
- 60g good-quality (70%)
- Dark chocolate chips

Instructions

- Oven preheat to 160 ° C (140 ° C fan / Gas 3). Line a large baking tray with a sheet of silicone or a parchment for baking.

- In a large bowl, combine the oats and the pecans. Heat the olive oil, butter, brown sugar, and rice malt syrup gently in a small non-stick pan until the butter has melted and the sugar and syrup dissolved. Do not let boil. Pour the syrup over the oats and stir thoroughly until fully covered with the oats.

- Spread the granola over the baking tray and spread out into the corners. Leave mixture clumps with spacing, instead of just spreading. Bake for 20 minutes in the oven until golden brown is just tinged at the edges. Remove from the oven and leave absolutely to cool on the tray.

- When it is cool, break with your fingers any larger lumps on the tray and then mix in the chocolate chips. Place the granola in an airtight tub or pot, or pour it. The granola is to last for at least 2 weeks.

Recipe 7: Sirty Blueberry Pancakes Ingredients

- Six bananas
- Six eggs
- tsp baking powder

- 1 2/3 cups rolled oats
- 1 1/2 cup blueberries
- ¼ teaspoon salt

Instructions

- Pop the oat flour in a high-speed blender and spin for 1 minute or until it has formed a flour of oats. Tip: make sure your mixer is dry before you do this or else it's all going to get soggy!

- Add the bananas, sugar, baking powder and salt to the blender and pump until forming a smooth batter for 2 minutes.

- Move the mixture and fold in the blueberries to a large pot. Leave the baking powder to rest for 10 minutes until it activates.

- To make your pancakes, add a dollop of butter to your frying pan over medium-high heat (this helps to make them very fluffy and crispy!).

- Add a couple of spoons of blueberry pancake mix and fry on the bottom side for until nicely golden. Toss the other side of the pancake to cook. You will Love it!

Recipe 8: Mocha Chocolate Mousse

Everyone likes chocolate, mousse. This one has a magnificent texture, light and airy. It's quick and simple to make, and best eaten the day after it's done.

- It serves 4–6

Ingredients

- 250g of dark chocolate (85% cocoa solids)
- Six medium free-range eggs, separated
- 4 tbsps. of strong black coffee
- 4 tbsp. almond milk
- Chocolate coffee beans (to decorate)

Instructions

- Firstly, you melt the chocolate over a pan of gently simmering water in a large bowl, ensuring the bowl 's bottom doesn't touch the water. Remove from heat the bowl and allow the melted chocolate to cool to room temperature.
- Once the melted chocolate has reached room temperature, whisk one at a time in the egg yolks and then fold gently in the coffee and almond milk.
- Whisk the egg whites with a handheld electric mixer until steep peaks form, then add a few tablespoons into the chocolate mixture to loosen it. Fold in the rest gently, using a large metal spoon.
- Move the mousse to single glasses and soften the color. Cover for at least 2 hours, ideally overnight, with a cling film and chill. Until serving, decorate with chocolate coffee beans.

Chapter 4: Benefits of Sirtfood and Meal Plan

4.1 What are the Health Benefits of Sirtfoods?

The sirtfoods are having a bundle of benefits for one's health besides weight loss. These health benefits will make your point clear about choosing these enriched food items. You are familiar with all the sirtfoods, let's discuss their benefits that you can get.

Parsley

Parsley has a lot of resources to sell than people expect. A 1/2 cup of fresh, chopped parsley provides:

- Calories: 11
- Carbs: 2 g
- Protein: 1 g
- Fat: minus 1 gram
- Fiber: 1 g
- Vitamin A: Reference Daily Intake (RDI) at 108 percent
- Vitamin C: RDI is 53 percent
- Vitamin K: RDI at 547 percent
- Folate: RDI's 11 per cent
- Potassium: RDI 4 per cent

Improves Bone Health

The herb is rich in many vitamins, especially vitamin K, essential for blood clotting and bone health. Parsley contains numerous antioxidant compounds that can support your wellbeing.

Your bones need varying amounts of specific vitamins and minerals to keep them safe and solid. Parsley is filled with vitamin K, which is a crucial nutrient for bone health. An incredible 547 per cent of RDI is given by a 1/2 cup (30 grams).

Vitamin K helps to build stronger bones by supporting cells called osteoblasts which strengthen bones. This vitamin also activates certain proteins which increase the density of bone minerals. Bone density is of utmost importance because a lower bone mineral density is linked with an increased risk of breakage, especially in older adults. Several studies indicate consuming high-vitamin K foods may reduce the risk of fractures. One study showed that higher intakes of vitamin K were associated with a 22 percent lower fracture risk. Typical intakes of vitamin K in the diet may be below the amounts required to enhance the bone mineral density and decrease the chances of fractures. Eating foods such as parsley can thus support bone health.

Parsley has Antioxidant Properties.

Antioxidants are compounds that prevent molecules from causing cell damage, called free radicals. For maintaining optimum health (6Trusted Source), your body needs a healthy balance of antioxidants and free radicals.

The major antioxidants in parsley are:

- Flavonoids

- Carotenoids

- Vitamin C

The herb is rich in a class of flavonoids known as antioxidants. The two principal flavonoids are myricetin and apigenin. Studies show that diets rich in flavonoids, including colon cancer, type 2 diabetes, and heart disease, may reduce your risk for conditions.

Beta-carotene and lutein are also two antioxidants, known as carotenoids. Many studies link higher carotenoid intake with lower risk for certain diseases, including lung cancer. Vitamin C also has significant antioxidant effects and plays a vital role in the promotion of immune health and chronic disease defense. Interestingly, dried parsley in antioxidants may be higher than the fresh sprigs. Also, one study found the dried herb contained 17 times more antioxidants than its fresh counterpart.

It Reduces the Chances of Cancer

Parsley is rich in vitamin C and flavonoid antioxidants which reduces your body's oxidative stress and reduces your risk of certain cancers. For example, a high intake of flavonoids in the diet can reduce the risk of colon cancer by up to 30 percent.

It Improves Your Vision

Lutein, beta-carotene, and zeaxanthin are three parsley carotenoids that help protect your eyes and promote good vision. Carotenoids are found in plants that have strong antioxidant activity. Lutein and zeaxanthin can prevent age-related macular degeneration (AMD), incurable eye disease and a leading cause of blindness around the world. Eating foods that are rich in lutein and zeaxanthin can reduce your risk of late AMD by up to 26%. Beta-carotene is another carotenoid that encourages healthy skin. This carotenoid in your body can be transformed to vitamin A. This beta carotene conversion explains why the parsley is so high in vitamin A. A 1/2 cup (30 grams) of freshly chopped leaves gives this vitamin 108 percent of the RDI.

Bird's Eye Chili

It is famous for reducing weight. These play an essential role in boosting the body's metabolism. The body temperature is raised as a result of this.

For getting the body back to its original temperature state, more calories will be consumed, thus increasing the metabolic process. Increased metabolism is beneficial and would increase the use of the unused fats stored in different body parts. As you'd noticed, an increase in metabolism leads to more sweating, resulting in weight loss. Fast metabolism, proper digestion, and the elimination of waste will minimize the body's chances of fat accumulation. Capsaicin is the chemical compound present in bird chili which results in burning sensation. The effects of this compound can vary from individual to individual. Many of them, however, experience a burning mouth, throat and stomach sensation upon ingestion. Bird's eye chili consumption thus increases the metabolism and reduces body weight.

Buckwheat

- **It Improves Heart Health**

This grain-like seed helps reduce inflammation and lower levels of LDL, or "bad cholesterol," which are both critical for maintaining heart health. Rutin, a form of phytonutrient and antioxidant that helps regulate blood pressure and reduce cholesterol, is the primary nutrient that provides these cardiovascular benefits.

- **Reduces Blood Sugar**

This pseudo cereal is very small on the glycemic index relative to other whole grains – this means that the carbohydrate content is absorbed gradually into the bloodstream, ensuring a constant supply of energy for the body. This nutritious seed helps with diabetes control by preventing a sudden spike in blood sugar and can boost insulin resistance.

- **It is Gluten Free and Non-Allergenic**

While this seed may be used in the same way as whole grains such as wheat and barley, it is naturally gluten-free, making it a better option for people with celiac disease or grain allergy.

- **Rich in Dietary Fiber**

This food contains 6 grams of dietary fiber for each cup serving of cooked groats. Dietary fiber helps keep food moving quickly across the digestive tract, which can make you stay fuller longer – that can be an advantage if you want to lose weight. It is also anti-cancer.

- **A Good Source of Vegetarian Protein**

This food is not only rich in vitamins and minerals but is also an excellent source of digestible plant protein. The diet contains as many as 14 grams of protein for every 100 grams of serving, and 12 separate amino acids to promote growth and muscle synthesis. The protein content is not as high as some beans and legumes, but it is higher than most whole grains.

- **Walnuts**

Walnuts have significant quantities of antioxidants in them that keep the immune system healthy and prevent the disease from occurring. Walnuts are the own vacuum cleaners because they sweep up countless bugs in the digestive system. The snack food, as a declared superfood because of its nutrient content, is also suitable for heart health and weight loss.

- **Rich in Omega-3 Fatty Acids**

The omega-3 fatty acids in walnuts are good for the brain as well. Having food rich in omega-3 fatty acids keeps the nervous system running smoothly, and the memory improves. These are also anti-cancer.

One serving of walnuts is 1 ounce or about seven walnuts. A serving of walnuts has:

- 185 calories
- 2.5 grams of monounsaturated fat
- 1.7 grams of saturated fat
- 4.3 grams of protein
- 1.9 grams of fiber
- 3.9 of carbohydrates
- 0.7 grams of sugar

Walnuts are fiber-rich and are a perfect way to keep the digestive system running properly. All humans daily need fiber to keep their intestines working correctly. Popular protein sources, such as meat and dairy products, are typically deficient in fiber. Having walnuts every day will help with digestive problems and keep your intestines working correctly.

- **Kale**

Kale is made of fibrous material, and therefore, like most leafy greens, it is excellent for digestion and elimination aid. One big tip is eating the stems, which contain a high amount of prebiotics, probiotic food in your microbiome.

- **Red Onion**

One cup of chopped onion contains approximately:

- 64 calories

- 15 grams of carbohydrate

- 0 grams of fat

- 3 grams of fiber

- 2 grams of protein

- 0 grams of cholesterol

- 7 grams of sugar

- 10% or more of the daily value for vitamin C, vitamin B-6 and manganese.

They also contain small amounts of calcium, iron, folate, magnesium, phosphorus and potassium and the antioxidants quercetin and sulfur. Raw onion is known to lower LDL (bad cholesterol) production and keep the heart-healthy. Vitamin C (which remains intact while in the raw form) together with the phytochemicals in the onions help to build immunity. Quercetin, a powerful compound found in onions, is suggested to play a role in cancer prevention, especially stomach and colorectal cancers. Chromium, which is also found in this root vegetable, may help to control blood sugar. It is said that a mixture of onion juice and honey (which helps make it less pungent) is effective as a treatment for fever, common cold, allergies, etc. In onions, folate also helps with depression and improves sleep and appetite. Vitamin C is helping to form collagen, which is responsible for the health of the skin and hair. Onions have proved their antibacterial and anti-inflammatory properties. One research has indicated that these antibacterial agents had freshly chopped raw onions, not chopped onions that have been left to sit for a day or two. Raw onion chewing improves our oral health (although your breath can stink). They help eliminate bacteria that may cause problems with tooth decay and gum.

- **Cocoa**

Together with Red Wine, dark chocolate has captured the most significant attention among the top 20 sirtfoods. Cocoa is rich in a particular group of polyphenols called flavonol, especially epicatechin, which is the actual sirtfood. In clinical trials, flavonol-rich cocoa has shown remarkable health benefits covering many of modern times' significant afflictions. It was particularly true in terms of heart health, where cocoa has shown promise to lower blood pressure, improve blood flow to the heart, prevent blood clots and reduce inflammation. Benefits can also be extended to aid in disease prevention, such as diabetes and cancer, and memory performance may be increased.

- **Medjool Dates**

The Medjool dates contain just about 66 calories each. They are an excellent fiber source and contain high levels of essential minerals, potassium, magnesium, copper, and manganese. Most do provide a substantial amount of fruit sugar, but that can make them an excellent alternative to more caloric dessert. These are a popular food for nomadic travelers in the Middle East where they grow wild since they provide plenty of energy and healthy nutrients with the added benefit of being readily available.

- **Strawberries**

Fiber is a necessity for healthy digestion and, naturally, strawberries contain about 2 g per serving. Problems that can result from fiber shortages include constipation and diverticulitis that is an inflammation of the intestines that affects around 50 per cent of people over 60. Fiber can also help combat type 2 diabetes. One of the best defenses against type 2 diabetes and heart disease is maintaining a healthy weight, not to mention just plain good for your overall wellbeing. "The strawberries are naturally low in calories (about 28 calories per serving), fat-free and low in both sodium and sugar," Edwards says. "Strawberries contain natural sugars, although total sugars are relatively low at 4 grams per serving — and the total content of carbohydrates is equivalent to less than half a slice of bread.

- **Extra Virgin Olive Oil**

In comparison, the natural extraction process used to manufacture Extra Virgin Olive Oil ensures it preserves all of the olive fruit's nutrients and antioxidants. It contains in particular over 30 different types of phenolic compounds which are powerful antioxidants that help protect the body from free radicals.

Free radicals are molecules which cause damage to cells and contribute to disease and ageing processes. Extra Virgin Olive Oil's fat composition is also a significant contributor to its healthiness. It consists predominantly of monounsaturated fat (about 73 per cent), a heart safe fat that is a staple of the Mediterranean diet. Studies consistently associate a diet high in monounsaturated fat with beneficial effects on cardiovascular disease indicators (heart disease and stroke). It involves raising indicators of chronic inflammation, blood pressure, levels of cholesterol and blood glucose. The Extra Virgin Olive Oil antioxidants are so resistant to high heat that they do not break down and end up being absorbed by the cooked food instead. It also helps the cooked food to retain certain nutrients which are usually lost by cooking.

Celery is rich in antioxidants that help remove free radicals from your cells which promote cancer. Celery extract was studied for two potential compounds of anticancer: apigenin, and luteolin. Apigenin disrupts free radicals in the body and can lead to death in cancer cells. It also seems to be promoting autophagy, a process in which your body removes dysfunctional cells or components that help prevent disease. Research also suggests luteolin, a celery-based plant flavonoid, could be responsible for its potential anticancer effects.

Researchers observed in one study that supplementation with luteolin decreased tumor levels of the mice by nearly half. And it slowed the tumors remaining to progress.

And if that's not enough, China studies say that eating two stalks a week could reduce the risk of lung cancer by up to 60%.

Other research suggests eating celery can be useful in combating breast, ovary, pancreas, liver and prostate cancers.

Celery is full of insoluble fiber, which can increase satiety and weight loss aid as well as helps in regularity. In other words, it can protect and treat constipation and help purify your bowels. Researchers looked into the effect of celery extract on the treatment of stomach ulcers in a 2010 report. And they examined its overall protective advantages on rat gastrointestinal system. Rats that had been pretreated with celery extract before they developed stomach ulcers experienced far less stomach damage than those that had not been pretreated. The researchers suggest this is likely because of the celery's antioxidant properties, a conclusion echoed in other celery and health studies.

- **Matcha Green Tea**

Like other green teas, Matcha contains a class of antioxidants named catechins. Matcha is high in an EGCG (epigallocatechin gallate) catechin, which is believed to have cancer-fighting effects on the body. Studies have linked green tea with a range of health benefits, such as helping protect heart disease, type-2 diabetes, cancer, and even promoting weight loss. Remember, that much of this research does not come from clinical trials that show green tea provides a benefit. Studies show the association between tea and better health, but it has not yet been proven causal.

- **Coffee**

Coffee is one of the best beverages in the world. It also tends to be relatively stable due to its high levels of antioxidants and beneficial nutrients. Coffee drinkers have a low risk of multiple serious illnesses.

That is because it contains a stimulant called caffeine — the psychoactive substance most commonly consumed in the world.

The caffeine is absorbed into the bloodstream when you drink a cup. It travels from there into your brain.

Caffeine blocks the inhibitory adenosine neurotransmitter within the brain. When this happens, the number of other neurotransmitters such as norepinephrine and dopamine increases, leading to increased neuron firing. Many controlled human studies show that coffee improves various aspects of brain function, including memory, mood, watchfulness, energy levels, reaction times and general mental function.

- **Turmeric**

One of the central claims to fame of turmeric is that it is commonly used to fight inflammation, and can be credited to turmeric for the bulk of the inflammation-fighting powers of turmeric. Curcumin may be a more effective anti- inflammatory treatment in the correct dose than conventional inflammation-fighting medicines. Curcumin is a safe and effective long-term treatment choice for people with osteoarthritis (OA), due to its potent anti-inflammatory properties. It also prevents heart diseases as well as diabetes type-2. It helps in delaying and reversing Alzheimer's disease. It helps in treating depression. It plays a role in treating rheumatoid arthritis.

Soy:

Only 10 percent -15 percent of total soybean fat is saturated. Many soy fats are polyunsaturated, including essential fats made from omega-6 and omega-3. It can be good for your heart as part of a healthy diet and may lower the risk of other diseases.

Soy foods are naturally cholesterol-free, as are all vegetables and grains.

Capers:

These savory herbs are vitamin storehouses such as vitamin A, vitamin K, niacin, and riboflavin.

Vitamin A enhances vision and helps us see in the night. It may also reduce the chances of certain cancers.

This vital vitamin helps our body to fight off infection and keeps our immune system. Vitamin K plays a crucial part in the health of bones. It lowers the risk of clotting blood. Niacin protects against cardiovascular diseases and thus aids executive functions, the nervous and digestive system. Riboflavin, also known as vitamin B2, helps the body turn food into fuel which keeps us healthy. Supporting the adrenal function is also well established. Thus it helps to keep the nervous system healthy. Capers are powerful fiber sources. Fiber cuts down on constipation. A capers tablespoon contains 0.3 grams of fiber, around 3 per cent of your daily minimum recommended intake of fiber.

4.2 Meal Plan and Weight Maintenance

We discussed about the phases of sirtfood diet briefly, now we will discuss in further details. The diet is subdivided into two phases. Phase 1 is called the 'hyper success phase' of 7 days, incorporating a Sirtfood-rich diet with mild calorie restriction, and Phase 2 is the 'maintenance phase' of 14 days, where you maintain your weight loss without reducing calories. Intake of calories is limited to 1,000 calories over the first three days (so, even more than on a five ratio two fasting day). The diet consists of 3 green juices rich in sirtfood and one meal rich in sirtfood and two squares of dark chocolate. Calories are increased to 1,500 calories over the remaining four days, and the diet includes two sirtfood-rich green juices and two sirtfood-rich meals each day. You are not permitted to drink any alcohol during Phase 1, but you are free to drink soda, tea, coffee and green tea. Phase 2 is not about limiting calories. Each day includes three sirtfood-rich meals and one green juice, plus one or two Sirtfood bite snacks, if necessary. You can drink red wine in Phase 2 but in moderation (recommendation is 2-3 glasses of red wine per week), as well as beer, tea, coffee, and green tea.

You are Wondering about the Meal Plan of Sirtfoods. Then here it comes. The Sirtfood Diet is not intended as a one-off 'diet' but rather as a way of life. You are advised to continue consuming a diet rich in Sirtfoods after you've completed the first three weeks and continue to drink your daily green juice. The writers of The Sirtfood Diet have continued to release The Sirtfood Diet Recipe Book since they released their initial book, with recipes for loads of more sirtfood-rich main meals, as well as recipes for alternatives to green juice and more hints and tips to adopt the Sirtfood Diet. There are also some Sirtfood dessert recipes here! The Sirtfood Diet authors recommend that phases 1 and 2 can be repeated if and when required for a health boost, or if things have gone a little off track. You can do this plan for up to two weeks, after which it's all about changing your lifestyle accordingly. There are no restrictions – aim to include as many sirt foods as you can in your diet, which will help your skin feel safer, healthier and smarter.

4.3 A Complete Seven Day Meal Plan for Sirtfood Diet Day One

- Three sirtfood green juices that may be of kale or grape and melon juice
- Two sirtfood bites (you can substitute these for 15-20g of dark chocolate if you wish)
- One sirtfood meal like I discussed the recipe of Kale and Red Onion Dhal with Buckwheat.

Day Two

- Three sirtfood green juices
- Two sirtfood bites
- One sirtfood meal for example baked salmon

Day 3

- Three sirtfood green juices
- Two sirtfood bites (Sirtfood dark chocolate bites)
- One sirtfood meal (Chargrilled Beef with a Red wine jus, Onion rings, Garlic kale and Herb roasted Potatoes)

Day 4

- Two sirtfood green juices
- Two sirtfood meals (1. Turmeric Chicken and Kale Salad with Dressing of Honey Lime and 2. Baked Chicken Breasts)

Day 5

- Two sirtfood green juices
- Two sirtfood meals (1. Prawn Arrabbiata, 2. Buckwheat Noodles with Chicken kale & Miso Dressing)

Day 6

- Two sirtfood green juices
- Two sirtfood meals (1. Strawberry Tabbouleh, 2. Asian King Prawn Stir Fry with Buckwheat Noodles)

Day 7

- Two sirtfood green juices
- Two sirtfood meals (1. Lamb, Butternut Squash and Date Tagine 2. Baked potatoes with spicy chickpea)

All the recipes are discussed in the second chapter. A day could look like this on a sirtfood diet:

- **Breakfast**

Mixed berries with soy yogurt, chopped walnuts and dark

chocolate

- **Lunch**

A sirtfood salad made with kale, parsley, celery, apple, olive oil walnuts mixed with lemon juice and ginger

- **Dinner**

Fried prawns with kale noodles and buckwheat.

The Sirtfood Diet is not intended as a one-off 'diet' but rather as a way of life. You are advised to continue consuming a diet rich in Sirtfoods after you've completed the first three weeks and continue to drink your daily green juice. The phases 1 and 2 can be repeated if required for a health boost if things have gone a little off track. However, after completing these phases, you are encouraged to continue "sirtifying" your diet by regularly incorporating sirtfoods into your meals. You can also include the sirt food in your diet as a snack or in the recipes you've already used. In this book, we have given a better compilation of Sirtfood recipes which can be followed. Furthermore, you are encouraged to continue drinking green juice every day. Thus the Sirtfood Diet becomes more a change in lifestyle than a one-time diet.

Should You Go for Sirtfood or Not?

The Sirtfood Diet supports fruit and vegetable consumption that detoxes your body to prevent harm. Many people are also attracted to the fact that you can eat chocolate and drink red wine in your diet! Hence it is advisable to turn to sirtfood diet, which is a new regime in diet foods. The 23 top Sirtfoods form the foundation of the Mediterranean diet and the Japanese diet, where obesity and disease inhabitants are lower. Five times as many foods is eaten in the Japanese as in the Western world.

It's important to identify healthy eating and exercise regimes that are practicable, do not take away from anything that you like and don't require you to practice throughout the week with an estimated 650 million obese adults worldwide. That's precisely what the Sirtfood diet does.

The idea is that certain foods activate the "skinny gene" paths, often triggered by fasting and workouts.

The best thing is that some foods and beverages, including dark chocolate and red wine, contain the chemicals known as polyphenols which activate the genes that imitate exercise and quickness.

Exercise during the first few weeks It would be sensitive to stop or reduce exercise during the first or two weeks of the diet, as your body sits to fewer calories. Hear your body and don't work out if you feel tired or have less energy than usual. Instead, make sure you continue to focus on principles for healthy lives such as appropriate daily concentrations of fiber, protein, fruit and vegetables. If you do practice, it is essential to eat protein, ideally one hour after your workout. When diet becomes a way of life Following exercise, protein repairs the muscles and can help relieve soreness. Several recipes include a protein that is ideal for post-exercise use such as sirt chili con carne, turmeric chicken and kale salad. You may try a sirt blueberry Smoothie if you wish something lighter and add some protein powder to add value. The type of fitness you do is yours, but exercises at home will allow you to make your choice of when to exercise, the kind of exercises that are convenient and short.

Sirtfood is a great way to change your eating habits, weight loss and a healthier feeling. The first few weeks can challenge you, but it's important to look for the most delicious foods to eat. In the first couple of weeks, be kind to yourself while your body adapts and exercise easily if you decide. If you're already a moderate or intense person, you could continue as you normally do, or administer your fitness according to your diet changes. As with any change in diet and practice, everything is about the person and how far you can go.

There's absolutely no reason you can't add a few sirtfoods to your food plan, Alpert says. "I think some really interesting things are here, like red wine, dark chocolate, matcha — these things I love," she says. "I love telling people what to focus on rather than nix off their diet." If it tastes indulgent and is healthy in small amounts, why not? Gans says she's a fan of many of the foods on the sirt list, including Mediterranean diet staples — the scientifically-backed gold standard for healthy eating — like olive oil, berries, and red wine. "I can get something rich in polyphenols and antioxidants behind foods," she says.

Blake agrees that the foods included in the diet have plenty to love, particularly the trendy ingredients such as turmeric and matcha that feel fresh and help make eating fun and interesting. "I see many plant-based foods that shine, and they're filled with phytonutrients," she said. "These are anti- inflammatory, and you're good at it."

However, all nutrition experts recommend rounding out the diet with some lean protein and healthy fats, including more nuts and seeds, avocado, and salmon-like fatty fish.

In addition to the kale and red onions, mix up your salad game with more types of veggies, spinach and roman lettuce. In the end? Some sirtfoods are A-OK for you to eat and safe, but don't swear to trigger that "skinny gene" by the diet yet.

If you follow this strategy, make sure to consume plenty of protein and change the food you eat to prevent deficiencies in vitamins. Take our pick? The diet is relatively strict. You are much better off cultivating a diet in the proportions that fit your individual needs to eat a variety of whole foods. If you still have questions that does it work. The et me remember you about the celebrities you used it.

Oh, it does according to their endorsements of other celebrities.

This book has inspiration from David Haye (Heavyweight Boxer), Lorraine Pascale (TV Chef and Food Writer), Jodie Kidd (Model), Sir Ben Ainslie (Olympic Gold Medalist) and a bundle of other celebrities. They all claim to have helped them lose weight, develop muscle and look fantastic.

Conclusion

There is a whole range of diets there to choose from, but it's all about doing what is right for you. Most of the people fed up of restricting all the food they love. They even do not get the desired results. The sirtfood diet, eating program stars like Adele and Pippa Middleton swear by, is one of the latest to gain popularity. The sirtfood diet is not restricting your chocolates and even allows you to take red wine. Sirtfood is high in nutrients that activate a so-called sirtuin gene. The "skinny gene" is activated when a lack of energy is generated after calories are restricted, said Goggins and Matten. You can reduce seven pounds in seven days yet in-taking a lot of green vegetables, nuts and drinks.

Sirtfood diet is divided into two phases. In the first phase, the calories are restricted to 1000 calories, and it is for seven days. In the second phase, you can take 1500 calories, and then four weeks of maintenance comes. The top most sirt foods include kale, celery, walnuts, Red wine, Strawberries, Onions, Soy, Parsley, Extra virgin olive oil, Dark chocolate (85% cocoa), Matcha green tea, Buckwheat, Turmeric, Arugula (rocket), Bird's eye chili, Lovage, Medjool dates, Red chicory, Blueberries, Capers and Coffee. The Sirtfood Diet has benefited including Pippa Middleton, Kim Cattrall and UFC World Champion Conor McGregor. You can consider these personalities as your motivation and lose weight without further delay. If you are concerned regarding your health, you need not worry, as all the foods on the list are going to benefit you. These are all having anti-inflammatory properties. These are good for your heart health, for your stomach, for your bones as well as your brain. Thus, now it's easy to burn the fat without wasting time on heavy exercises and waiting for months for the results. You only need to follow the simple recipes given and see the magic.